Complementary Health Therapies:
A GUIDE FOR NURSES
AND THE CARING PROFESSIONS

Edited by
DENISE F. RANKIN-BOX

CROOM HELM
London & Sydney

© 1988 Denise F. Rankin-Box
Croom Helm Ltd, Provident House,
Burrell Row, Beckenham, Kent BR3 1AT
Croom Helm Australia, 44–50 Waterloo Road,
North Ryde, 2113, New South Wales

British Library Cataloguing in Publication Data

Complementary health therapies: a guide
  for nurses and caring professions.
  1. Health 2. Nursing
  I. Rankin-Box, Denise F.
  613'.024613   RT67

  ISBN 0-7099-5008-X

Filmset by Mayhew Typesetting, Bristol, England
Printed and bound in Great Britain by
Biddles Ltd, Guildford and King's Lynn

Contents

Denise F. Rankin-Box, BA(Hons), SRN, DipTD, qualified as an SRN at Addenbrookes Hospital, Cambridge. Following work with the Flying Doctor Service in Australia and Voluntary Medical Work in Papua New Guinea, she returned to England and subsequently obtained an Honours degree in Sociology.

She is currently studying for a PhD in the Department of Nursing, University of Manchester.

She has a particular interest in complementary/holistic nursing and therapies on this topic, and in the use of Shiatsu within current nursing practice. She has been practising Shiatsu for four years and has conducted a number of workshops and short courses for nurses and other health care workers.

Contributors

Brian Butler, BA, Touch for Health Foundation, Faculty Member for Great Britain, Touch for Health Foundation, Surbiton, Surrey, UK.

Stephanie Downey, SRN, BA(Hons), BAc, Acupuncture Practitioner, Brighton Acupuncture Clinic, Brighton, Sussex, UK.

Hazel Goodwin, Practitioner and Teacher of Reflexology, Massage and Yoga, Brighton, Sussex, UK.

Neil Gulliver, Associate Teacher of the Kushi Institute, Shiatsu Society Registered Practitioner and Teacher, Ipswich, Suffolk, UK.

Allan Mason, BA, GradDipPhys, MCSP, DipTP, Department of Health Studies, Sheffield City Polytechnic, Sheffield, UK.

Jean Orr, MSc, BA, CNAA, SRN, HVTutCert, CertED, Lecturer in Nursing, University of Manchester, UK.

Chandra Patel, MD, MRCGP, Senior Clinical Lecturer, Department of Community Medicine, University College London and Middlesex Hospital Medical School, London, UK.

Denise F. Rankin-Box, BA(Hons), SRN, DipTD, Department of Nursing, University of Manchester, UK.

Janet Southall, SRN, DipBWOY, County Representative of TET (Teacher Education Tutor) for the British Wheel of Yoga, Middlesex, UK.

Jacques Tamin, MB, ChB, MRCGP, DRCOG, General Practitioner and Hypnotherapist, Greyland Medical Centre, Manchester, UK.

Sue Thame, BA, Teaching Member of Society of Teachers of the Alexander Technique. Recent Director of Alexander Teaching Associates.

Pat Turton, MMedSci, BSc, SRN, NDNCert, Lecturer in Nursing, University of Manchester, UK.

Acknowledgements

Grateful acknowledgements are given to the International Institute of Reflexology for permission to use their reproduction of an Egyptian Wall Painting (Chapter 5); and to Deborah Pleese for illustrating Figures 4.2 and 4.3 in Chapter 4.

I would like to thank all the contributors for their time, commitment and support in ensuring this book became a reality.

Special thanks to my husband, Dr Ian Rankin, for his support, and the many hours spent in discussions concerning holistic health care and its application within current medical and nursing practice; to Stephanie Downey for her friendship and shared enterprises within the field of complementary therapies, and to Liz Perkins for her insightful comments whilst the original ideas for this book became structured and honed down to its final form.

I am also grateful to Christine Garratt and Joyce Fernandes for their speed and efficiency in typing many parts of this manuscript.

Finally, on behalf of the contributors, I should like to thank all those who assisted in the compilation of these chapters as they went through various drafts.

Denise F. Rankin-Box

1

Introduction

Denise F. Rankin-Box

In recent years western models of health and illness, along with the role played by medicine and nursing, have been critically assessed. The belief that medicine, grounded in the natural sciences, provides the only means of mediating between people and disease is being increasingly questioned and there is a growing desire to explore alternative methods of health care which are both non-invasive and non-iatrogenic.

Many of those methods centre upon the concept of 'holism' an approach which highlights the interdependence of the physical, spiritual and environmental aspects of our lives. An imbalance in one or all three of these factors contributes to disease and ill health.

In his book *Holistic Living*, Patrick Pietroni describes the concept of holism as

> . . . essentially about an approach each one of us can use to help us understand ourselves and our place in the world in which we live. From this deeper understanding we can begin to make informal choices about our health and the way we conduct our lives.[1]

Holistic health, then, represents an approach to all aspects of life and has implications for each one of us, whether as a carer or as the recipient of care. It directs individuals towards a greater understanding of the way in which social, emotional, physical and spiritual aspects of our lives interrelate to influence personal wellbeing.

This issue is important because there is a possibility that the tide of enthusiasm breaking over complementary therapies may lead nurses and others involved in health care to assume that many holistic therapies represent yet another procedure to be learnt or

1

another task to be fitted into one's time in an already overstretched schedule.

An holistic approach to nursing implies a shift in our perception of current health practices. While the recipients of care are referred to as patients, in a number of chapters, mainly for the sake of familiarity or convenience, it may be more appropriate to regard them as clients since this label implies a shift in approach towards nursing care. Emphasis is placed upon the sharing of decision-making and the setting up of acceptable goals for both client and practitioner rather than on treating patients. In order to do this, sharing information and education is viewed as a fundamental basis of therapy, and the client is encouraged to take responsibility for his or her own health or ill-health, towards preventing further disorders.

WESTERN MEDICINE AND THE HOLISTIC APPROACH

Western medicine has so far attempted to treat the body systematically and organically 'like a machine that could be understood in terms of its parts . . . (Stephanie Downey in Chapter 2 of this book, p. 8). While this approach is not to be underrated, in practice it frequently minimises the impact of many broader or more insidious factors in our lives that can have serious implications for our health.

Stephanie Downey also notes (Chapter 2 of this book, p. 8) that, 'the recognition that our bodies, minds and spirits are all related and affect each other is not new, but in western medicine, the emergence of the scientific revolution initiated the reductionist approach to health care'.

What would appear to be new, however, is the increasing interest shown by many orthodox practitioners of western medicine and nursing who have become aware that the reductionist approach to health care is not proving to be the panacea for all ills. In the search for an improved medical system, western medicine is now acknowledging a range of frequently well established forms of health care approaches practised in other cultures and derived from various philosophical origins.

NURSING AND HOLISM

The search for an improved model of medical care has also extended to nursing practice where many nurses are disillusioned with the current approach to health. Despite models of nursing advocating care of patients on both a psychosocial and spiritual level, low staffing numbers and increased workloads frequently inhibit such a total care approach. Concerns have been raised that some nursing practices only contribute to relieving symptoms rather than the underlying problems that many patients face. Consequently staff may feel that neither they nor the patient benefit greatly from the interaction. The demands upon nurses in this type of environment produces its own stresses, and terms such as 'burnout' are becoming increasingly common. As a result, along with doctors, nurses are developing a greater interest in therapies that not only direct themselves towards care of the 'whole' person, but also regard health of the nurse as an important factor in successful treatment.

Holistic nursing is a phrase which has found its way from America, but it is not necessarily the same as a problem-solving approach to individualised patient care. Although there is some common ground there are basic philosophical differences. For example, while the term 'patient' is used in this text for familiarity it does imply a certain passivity of role. We do things *for* a patient and too rarely *with* the patient.

Holistic care recognises the interplay of mind, spirit and body which is consistent with many current nursing theories, and in this respect it has much in common with orthodox nursing practice where the aim is to treat patients as 'whole' people.

As Pam Holmes states, this theme is promoted during nurse training,

> Nursing schools teach that total nursing care demands the nurse assesses and responds to patients on every level of his/her being — political, social, psychological, religiously and physically. An holistic approach is the corner stone of both nursing and alternative therapies.[2]

Despite such an ideal picture it would seem that with rapidly increasing demands placed upon nurses today, in terms of lower staffing levels, the extended role of the nurse and the continuous pressure of long waiting lists cause increasing alienation from the whole patient.

Given the need to stretch financial and nursing resources, priorities are being set which perhaps, like their medical counterparts, put nursing on the road to becoming disease-oriented — seeing patients as malfunctioning organs rather than as people. With these problems it is initially hard to envisage how complementary therapies and an holistic approach to nursing care can improve the situation. .

A central factor in holistic nursing depends equally upon *what* one does when with a patient and *how* it is done. It is essential to acknowledge that such an approach to patient care interprets health and illness equally in relation to every aspect of the *nurse's* life as well as that of the patient's — whether physical, spiritual or emotional.

Holistic care focuses upon the interdependence between client and practitioner — on sharing power, information and responsibility, exchanging views and comments and actively engaging patients in their own recovery. Emphasis is on the whole rather than the symptom; it is also fundamental that the person becomes involved and responsible for his/her own body — a factor that current western medicine is perhaps only just beginning to acknowledge.

Such an approach shifts the focus of care from the treatment of sickness towards the prevention of illness and what has been called a state of 'positive health'. Although this concept is arguably not new, the term 'prevention' broadens the concept of caring for the sick to include the maintenance of health in both patient and practitioner — highlighted by the maxim of the British Holistic Medical Association (BHMA): 'Physician Heal Thyself'.

Complementary therapies offer nursing an alternative approach to current practice by seeking to promote the health of the nurse as well as of those in their care. While this latter issue is of growing concern it would seem that unless health workers are prepared to review their own approach to health, there is a risk that complementary therapies will be offered to patients as just another procedure, another task.

COMPLEMENTARY OR ALTERNATIVE THERAPIES?

The concept of 'holism' has been referred to throughout this introduction with particular reference to 'complementary therapies'. Many of these practices have also been labelled 'alternative'. However, the terms 'complementary' and 'alternative' are conceptually distinct and should *not* be used interchangeably.

The *Oxford English Dictionary* defines 'alternative' as the process of 'excluding one thing in favour of another'. 'Complementary', however, embodies the idea of coexistence and enhancement and is referred to in the dictionary as 'of two or more things mutually complementing each other's deficiencies'. It would seem that the word 'alternative' is both misleading and contains a certain irony when one considers that many unorthodox therapies have been practised for hundreds of years — and in the case of shiatsu, acupuncture and therapeutic touch, thousands of years. In this respect perhaps western medicine is the alternative practice.

Consequently, use of the term 'complementary' is preferred as it would seem to be the most accurate definition or umbrella under which to place the therapies described here, since each has the potential to complement and enhance current nursing and medical practice.

THE THERAPIES

The aim of this book is to introduce the interested nurse or other health professional to a range of therapies which can be integrated into general health care. A common bond unites each therapy in that they all attempt in varying ways to draw upon the self-healing capacity of the body to promote a return to health and help the individual to 'adapt more harmoniously with their surroundings'.[3]

Health is regarded as relatively unique to each individual, dependent upon his/her lifestyle, and is also taken to include not only the absence of symptoms but a complete state of physical and mental wellbeing (as defined by the World Health Organization). Central to any form of care is the ability to communicate whether by touch, close proximity to someone, massage, or verbal and non-verbal interaction. While this aspect is regarded as fundamental to many of the therapies described here, it was felt that the inclusion of a chapter expressly on social skills could help to address a number of concerns and difficulties that staff may encounter during their daily work. Too often social skills are regarded as inherent abilities possessed by all rather than skills to be learnt and refined. Consequently, an awareness of methods that may enhance the communication process is valuable to both orthodox and complementary perspectives of health care.

The contributors in this book are all practitioners in their respective fields, and with the exception of acupuncture all the therapies described are non-invasive and may be taught to patients to generate self-care.

In each chapter the author sets out to describe the philosophy behind a therapy and its applications within health care and nursing. Where possible, research findings are cited and references given. However, the number of studies given should not be interpreted as proof that a therapy does or does not work.

First, there is considerable debate regarding what constitutes an appropriate research method to investigate therapies that care for the whole person. While certain quantitative measurements may be recorded in some instances, this approach is not viable when attempting to evaluate the spiritual and emotional aspects of treatment said to occur *simultaneously* with any physical care given.

Second, there is an unwillingness to fund research given the absence of an appropriate research methodology. Linked to this is an awareness that such funding would not necessarily have any commercial or profit-making repercussions for many companies, for example, in terms of drugs or medication. As Fulder states:[3]

> The total number of published, objective, controlled, clinical studies on the effectiveness of chiropractic, osteopathy, healing, naturopathy, homeopathy, Alexander Technique, radionics and massage *put together*, is no more than the number usually required to put a minor new drug on the market . . .

In publishing a small selection of the therapies that have the potential for complementing or enhancing current nursing and medical health care, it is hoped that readers will be encouraged to learn more about various topics, attend courses and learn how to implement them within daily health care. Complementary therapies are not another bandwagon, another nursing task or 'fad'. The philosophies underlying many of these therapies offer something else. In the words of Michio Kushi: 'Instead of complexity, they offer simplicity. Abandoning the artificial, they stress the natural. The purpose is to unite the scientific knowledge that modern man has acquired with the intuitive knowledge that man once enjoyed'.[4]

REFERENCES

1. Pietroni P. *Holistic Living: A Guide to Self-Care* (J.M. Dent and Sons Ltd, London, 1986), p. 1.

2. Holmes P. 'Holistic Nursing', *Nursing Times*, 18 April 1984, pp. 28–9.

3. Fulder S. *The Handbook of Complementary Medicine* (Coronet Books, London, 1984).
4. Kushi M. Leaflet. (The Michio Kushi Institute of Great Britain, London, 1981).

For the sake of simplicity the pronoun 'he' is used throughout this book and should be taken to mean female or male.

USEFUL ADDRESSES

British Holistic Medical Association
179 Gloucester Place
London
NW1 6DX
Telephone: 01 262 5299 or 01 402 2768
(Information on holistic and complementary medicine; membership open to the public)

Council for Complementary and Alternative Medicine
Suite 1
19a Cavendish Square
London
W1M 9AD
Telephone: 01 409 1440

Research Council for Complementary Medicine
Suite 1
19a Cavendish Square
London
W1M 9AD
Telephone: 01 493 6930
(Coordinates and promotes research)

College of Health
18 Victoria Park Square
London
E2 9BR
Telephone: 01 980 6263

Community Health Foundation
188–194 Old Street
London
EC1V 9BP
Telephone: 01 252 4076
(Runs various classes, workshops; associated with East/West Centres Michio Kushi Institute)

Michio Kushi Institute
188 Old Street
London
EC1
Telephone: 01 251 4076

2

Acupuncture

Stephanie Downey

INTRODUCTION

The growing popularity of 'alternative' medicine in the West clearly indicates the increasing dissatisfaction with modern scientific medicine and the urgent need to find new approaches to health and illness. Much of the attraction of these unorthodox forms of treatment is due to their holistic philosophies based on the principle of the whole body: the recognition that our bodies, minds and spirits are all related and affect each other. In other cultures this concept is commonplace, but in western Europe it is relatively new.

Since the rise of science from the 15th century onwards, western medicine has increasingly treated the human body as a machine that could be understood in terms of its parts. Disease is 'caused' by a biological malfunction that can be isolated and corrected with drugs or surgery. Athough this reductionist approach has had considerable success on the chemical and structural levels, it obviously neglects major aspects of human behaviour that influence our state of health. As a result of this gap in western medicine and the absence of a new model of health care, there has been little choice but to reconsider those already well-established 'holistic' medical systems, either revived from the past (such as homeopathy and herbalism), or taken from other cultures.

Acupuncture, as an example of the latter comes from a long tradition of eastern philosophy, and consequently has very differing perceptions of health and illness. The question is, how far can such an archaic and culturally alien system of medicine be relevant to us today? Attempts *are* being made to answer this question and to incorporate these approaches to health into orthodox medicine,[1] but this has largely resulted in a clash of philosophies with the entrenched scientific medical model in total opposition to holistic ideals.

As well as looking at how acupuncture works, I want to consider what it has to offer orthodox western medicine; the dangers of being subsumed by the medical model; and how new perspectives are needed to overcome the obvious limitations of our present approach to illness, so that the needs of both practitioners and users of medical services can be more effectively met.

HISTORICAL BACKGROUND

Acupuncture originated in China during the Stone Age between 8000 and 3000 BC, and is a healing system that has been used and developed since then in many parts of the world. In China it is rarely practised on its own, but forms one part of a whole system of medicine that includes herbs, diet and exercise.

There is evidence that stone was used originally to puncture the skin; these primitive 'needles' were later refined to be made out of bone and bamboo. Metal needles, initially made of bronze, have been discovered dating back to 2205 BC, gold and silver have since been used, and by 200 BC steel was available.[2]

The theory of channels of energy with specific points along their courses is central to acupuncture. It has been widely debated which were discovered first, points or channels. However, the most popular view is that the points were noticed first through hundreds of years of observing spontaneously tender spots on the body and specific reactions to pressing or puncturing these points. Eventually, by 200 AD, all the points were known and a complex theoretical system of meridian pathways had been established.[3]

Modern acupuncture, both in China and the West, is based on theories about the function of the body which developed through a process of observation and experimentation over 8000 years. Around 100 BC this was ultimately formalised into a system of medicine in the 'Nei Jing', or The Yellow Emperor's Inner Classic of Chinese Medicine. Although acupuncture has grown and developed over the centuries, this has all taken place within the general framework established under the aegis of the Yellow Emperor.[4]

Acupuncture is currently practised in hospitals throughout China alongside modern western medicine, both contributing equally to the provision of health care. In recent years acupuncture is being used increasingly in the West in both hospitals and the community. Its effectiveness has been recognised by the World Health Organization which advocates its use, and recognises its success in the treatment of 300 different diseases.[5]

ACUPUNCTURE: THEORY AND PHILOSOPHY

The aim of acupuncture is to correct imbalances of energy in the body through the insertion of needles into specific points, and so assist the body's own recuperative powers. Behind this deceptively simple premise lies a vast and complex body of knowledge, which reflects the underlying Chinese philosophy.

The concepts used in Chinese medicine to classify and explain the human body are the same as those used to describe the universe as a whole: the all-pervasive Qi (energy), the balance of Yin and Yang and the cyclical laws of the Five Elements. Fundamental to Chinese thought is the idea of both the macrocosm and the microcosm, where the human body is seen to reflect and obey the same laws as those that govern the universe as a whole. In this way the human organism is inseparable from the environment, and within the body there can be no understanding of the parts except in relation to the whole.

Qi and meridian pathways

Central to all Chinese medicine is the concept of Qi (also spelt Ki and Chi), something that has no western equivalent, but can broadly be defined as vital energy or life-force. Every living thing in the universe has Qi running through it. It is Qi that distinguishes a living being from an inanimate object, the quality and amount of Qi determining one's health and vitality. Its physical existence is given less importance than its function since Qi, like many aspects of Chinese medicine, is perceived by what it does rather than its structural composition. Its functions are basically to provide the source of movement in the body, to keep the blood circulating, to fight disease, and to warm the body.

Qi is distributed around the body through a network of interconnecting channels. Through superficial and internal pathways it goes deep to the organs and passes through different levels to just below the skin where it can be contacted with acupuncture needles.

There are 12 main meridians and eight extra meridians, all

Figure 2.1: The bladder meridian

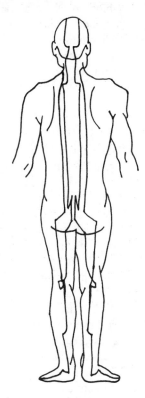

following fixed pathways to connect with the viscera, the sense organs, the four limbs and the skin. Of the main meridians there are six Yin and six Yang meridians, each named after an associated organ and paired, Yin with Yang:

Yin	*Yang*
Lung	Colon
Spleen	Stomach
Heart	Small intestine
Heart governor	Triple heater
Kidney	Bladder
Liver	Gallbladder

Illness occurs primarily when there is an excess, deficiency or stagnation of Qi either throughout the whole body or within a

11

specific organ or meridian. For example, pain and stiffness in the back may be caused by blocked Qi in the bladder meridian. This meridian goes down either side of the spine, down the legs to the little toe, so the back problem may be treated by using points on the bladder channel away from the affected area, for example on the leg, to help move the Qi and relieve the pain (Fig. 2.1).

Yin and Yang

Yin and Yang are relative terms, Yin representing all that is yielding, quiescent, slow, dark; and Yang symbolising dynamic, aggressive, fast-moving and expansive qualities. The interaction of these two primary and opposing forces is the means by which everything in the universe is produced. In the human body, Yin represents the interior, blood and organs, the lower part of the body, the front, slowness, cold, damp, heaviness, calmness, quiet, passivity, introspection. The Yang counterpart of these qualities are exterior, skin and flesh, the upper part of the body, the back, fast-moving, hot, dry, lightness, agitation, noise, action, extroversion.

Since health depends on Yin and Yang existing in equal proportions, illness is characterised by an excess or deficiency of either Yin or Yang. For example, a disease due to excess Yang may manifest suddenly, such as an acute headache, with disturbed vision, bloodshot eyes, red face, in a person prone to extreme outbursts of anger and shouting. The aim of treatment in this case would be to pacify the Yang and increase the Yin, to reach a more even state of balance.

Organs and their functions

Although the organs (and associated channels) in Chinese medicine have the same names as their counterparts in modern western medicine there is a vast difference between them. In the West we classify organs in terms of anatomical structures that are connected to one another through their specific physiologies, producing physical changes measured in biochemical or other quantifiable terms. Organs in Chinese medicine are important only for their functions, not their structures. The early Chinese doctors had no apparatus to see inside the body, and dissection was socially proscribed.[6] Consequently, through years of empirical observation the Chinese developed an elaborate theory of 'physiology' based purely on what they could observe, see, feel, smell, ask from the 'outside'. In this way, the state of an organ could be assessed by feeling the pulse, looking at the tongue and asking about all areas governed by that particular organ.

Chinese medicine recognises 12 organs, each one a functional system responsible for a specific physical, emotional and spiritual aspect of human life. For example, the liver's main function is the storage of blood and maintenance of free-flowing Qi throughout the body. It also governs the muscles and tendons, the eyes, and the nails; so any disturbance in these physical aspects may point to disharmony in the liver. In the area of emotions, the liver is related to anger and irritability and may be affected if these feelings are either excessive or suppressed. Its spiritual domain represents life drive or zest for living, the outward expansion from self to the universe, the ability to plan one's life. If the liver is imbalanced it could manifest as passivity, depression or lack of interest in life. Since Chinese philosophy views human beings as inseparable from the universe as a whole, the liver and all the organs also relate to the natural world. The liver corresponds to the element wood, the season spring, the climate wind and the colour green. Hay fever often stems from a liver imbalance as it commonly begins around spring, affects the eyes and is made worse by windy weather. In this system mind, body, spirit and environment are not disconnected parts but simply phenomena that exist along a continuum. Differences are of shade, not of kind.[7]

Five Elements

Where Yin and Yang explains the origin of the world, the theory of the Five Elements sets out to interpret the structure of the universe. Human existence is inextricably linked to the natural world — seasons, climates, elements, growth and decay. In the same way as the seasons change cyclically with the growth of spring rising to summer, sinking into the harvest of autumn and contraction of winter, so too does the human body undergo such changes and is governed by the laws of the Five Elements — *fire, earth, metal, water, wood* — which are arranged in a cycle of creation, moving clockwise. It is a cycle of transformation, beginning with wood and the season spring creating fire (summer), which then generates the element earth (Indian summer) to create metal (autumn) and so to transform into water and winter (Fig. 2.2).[8]

Figure 2.2: Cycle of transformation

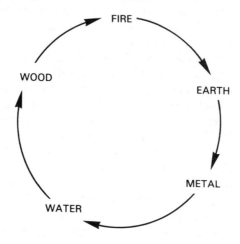

Figure 2.3: Cycle of control or destruction

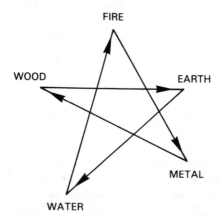

As well as creating one another through this clockwise movement, the Elements or transformations also have a cycle of control
or destruction (Fig. 2.3). Here wood controls the earth which
similarly checks the action of water; water destroys fire, fire
destroys metal and metal restrains wood.

Each element, as well as being related to a season, also
corresponds to a whole series of physical, mental and spiritual

qualities that include organs, tissues, smells, tastes, emotions and colours.

For example:

Metal : autumn; lungs/colon; skin; nose; grief; animal spirit (instinct)

Water : winter; bladder/kidneys; bones; ears; fear; willpower

Wood : spring; liver/gallbladder; tendons; eyes; anger; soul

Fire : summer; heart/small intestine; blood vessels; tongue; joy; spirit

Earth : late summer; spleen/stomach; flesh; mouth; pensiveness; intellect

By applying the laws of the Five Elements to the human body, each organ with its physical, emotional and spiritual dimension is connected to and affected by one another. Health is based on the delicate balance of energy within the Five Elements. If it is excessive or deficient in a certain area, the cycles of creation or control will break down resulting in physical or emotional ill-health. In such a way disharmony in one area will cause an imbalance somewhere else in the body.

PRACTICE: DIAGNOSIS AND TREATMENT

Where orthodox medicine practises differential diagnosis — a process of elimination to isolate single causes, in acupuncture the diagnosis is made by collecting as much information as possible to create a complete picture of a particular individual. Data is collected through the 'four methods' of diagnosis: asking, looking, listening/smelling and touching. A detailed case history is taken to place the person and his/her disharmony in its full context from macrocosm to microcosm. For example, *asking*: questions will refer to possible climatic and seasonal influences: wind, heat, damp, cold; living conditions; emotional states; all physical symptoms even if seemingly unrelated; diet; lifestyle; occupation; amount/type of exercise; sleep; past medical history, constitution, parents' health; drugs taken; past trauma, and anything else that the person may feel has an effect on his/her health.

Looking involves the observation of someone's general appearance, manner, facial colour, posture, state of the spirit — shine of the eyes, clarity of thought and responsiveness. The tongue will also be examined to determine from its colour, shape and coating the state of Qi, presence of heat, damp, cold, stagnation of energy, progression and degree of illness and in what part of the body.

The acupuncturist will *listen* to the strength of the voice, quality of respiration, and for the existence of any coughing.

Smelling is less important than it used to be, the tradition being that a smell of rancid meat indicates heat, a pungent/fishy smell indicates cold.

By *touching* one can feel for areas of heat or cold on the body or make an abdominal diagnosis, although the most important application of touch is in feeling the pulse. This refined diagnostic method which takes years to perfect involves feeling the radial artery in three positions on each wrist. Each position can be felt on two levels, the superficial pulse by pressing lightly, and the deeper pulse by pressing a little harder. Altogether this corresponds to six organs on each wrist, the Yin organs being felt at the deep position, and the Yang organs more superficially. It is possible to feel the rhythm, speed and quality of the pulse which tells the practitioner about the state of energy in different organs often before symptoms appear or before a person is even aware of any health problems.

The holistic tradition of Chinese medicine is such that no single part can be understood except in relation to the whole. The main emphasis is on the person as an individual within a unique social, physical, and emotional context. The aim is always not just to treat symptoms (although they will be dealt with) but to look beyond to causes which may go back many years and relate to any aspect of the person's lifestyle. Often changes can be made in areas such as diet and exercise to enhance and consolidate the treatment and to encourage the person to take an active part in the maintenance of his/her own health. Prevention has always been important to the Chinese, and traditionally doctors were only paid while their patients were healthy.[9]

USES OF ACUPUNCTURE

When asked what acupuncture can treat, it is important to stress that acupuncture treats *people* not diseases. Although several people may be diagnosed as suffering from arthritis in orthodox medicine, in acupuncture their conditions would all be seen and treated quite differently. Each person's arthritis is a consequence of a particular constitution, lifestyle, climatic influence, emotional response and dietary habit, so treatment will be directed to the *individual* picture of disharmony: 'Chinese Medicine can only meaningfully be presented in terms of a particular patient at a particular time'.[10]

Contrary to popular medical belief, acupuncture is not just a method of pain relief, but has over the centuries been treating a whole range of diseases.[11] It is especially valuable in chronic conditions that conventional treatment can only alleviate with drugs, for example: asthma, hay fever, sinusitis; hypertension; depression; painful conditions anywhere in the body such as headaches, migraine, arthritis, back pain, stiffness of joints or muscles.

Many acute cases can also be treated including strains and sprains, shingles, cystitis, menstrual disorders, diarrhoea and vomiting, coughs, colds and sore throats. In China today many major diseases are treated in hospital using acupuncture, such as kidney stones, gallstones, coronary diseases, strokes, pancreatitis, appendicitis and diabetes. Acpuncture also recognises and treats many disharmonies that have no medical diagnosis, a non-specific 'not quite right' feeling, characterised by any of the following: tiredness, lethargy, vague aches and pains, digestive problems, difficulty in sleeping, anxiety, tension, palpitations or dizziness.

Finally, acupuncture is being increasingly used to help reduce withdrawal symptoms in cases of addiction. Many acupuncturists have experienced a growing demand from those who need help in reducing their dependency on alcohol, cigarettes or drugs. This is also an area that has attracted the attention of the medical profession and there has been a significant amount of media coverage recently, describing doctors who had begun to use acupuncture techniques in their work with drug addicts (for example, in the recently established centre in Liverpool for the treatment of heroin addiction). However, a serious problem is emerging: the appropriation of acupuncture by western medicine (similarly demonstrated in the use of acupuncture analgesia), where it is practised in a limited way *without fully understanding its extent and scope as a medical system.*

As a medical system acupuncture is safe, effective and cheap. Although it is no cure-all, and certainly could not compete with modern scientific medicine in many acute life-threatening cases, it has a definite part to play in future health care provision both in China and the West.

However, if it is to be truly viable, the theory of acupuncture really needs to adapt and incorporate the additional hazards of our modern western lifestyles, as recognised by Dubos: 'The social, economic and political complexities of modern industrial society have created an environment which is in many ways hostile to the biological and psychological integrity of its inhabitants.'[12]

ACUPUNCTURE TODAY

Athough the ancient theories of acupuncture are still valid, it cannot be denied that the pressures of life in ancient China were probably very different from those we experience today. Many modern social and environmental factors have an increasing influence over our health and need to be acknowledged: the effects of pollution, chemicals, food additives, pesticides; chronic emotional problems and stress; long-term medication, such as steroids, aspirin, antibiotics: 'pleasure drugs', stimulants, tea, coffee, tobacco, alcohol, plus the effects of X-rays, vaccinations, anaesthetics and operations.[13]

The philosophy and theory behind Chinese medicine is essentially holistic, and it is important that this should be maintained in practice. Unfortunately this ideal is often difficult to uphold, and situations arise where acupuncture is practised in a way that closely resembles the orthodox version, namely the 'active' doctor–'passive' patient relationship. Although acupuncture is a progressive therapy in that it recognises mind/body interactions and attempts to stimulate the body's own self-healing abilities, if it is to develop as a viable health system of the future and avoid the pitfalls of modern western medicine, it must be more than just a technique of inserting needles into specific points. Acupuncture, and any medicine that aspires to holistic treatment needs to work on three levels.

Diagnosis and treatment by a health practitioner

This is the most basic and traditional method. It is valid, although on its own encourages dependence, takes power and responsibility away from the patient, and often mystifies the whole area of health.

Education, self-help, advice and referral

The aim here is to recognise the uniqueness of the individual, to encourage him/her to be involved in his/her own particular illness, and as far as possible to take responsibility for improving health.

This may be either on an individual level or in the form of support groups, both of which give back some control to the person concerned. Advice may be given regarding changes in diet, exercise, relaxation or emotional adjustments, depending on the skill of the practitioner. One should always be aware of the limitations of a specific treatment and suggest referrals to other therapies where appropriate. There are so many different approaches to health it is unlikely that any one has the ability to be totally holistic.

Socioeconomic factors

Health cannot be considered purely as an individual problem isolated from other issues such as income, lifestyle, education, nutrition. The roots of many diseases can be traced back to these factors, and if any progress is to be made it is vital that research is directed towards these wider areas to expose general patterns of ill-health, who is affected most and why. Preventive medicine is not just something to be practised by individuals, but must take place on a social level as well.

ACUPUNCTURE FOR NURSES AND HEALTH PRACTITIONERS

Since it takes at least three years' training to be a qualified acupuncturist, it cannot easily be incorporated into nursing as a supplementary skill, in the same way as massage or shiatsu for example. However, many nurses disillusioned by the limitations of their roles within the health system yet still wishing to remain in health care, are choosing to broaden their skills by taking an additional training in some kind of complementary medicine. Within the existing structure, there are at the moment two clear openings for the nurse/acupuncturist: in maternity units, and in occupational health.

In maternity units

An increasing number of women are looking for alternatives to drug-oriented childbirth. Along with hypnotherapy, acupuncture has been used successfully to give pain relief during labour. At the moment acupuncturists are usually contracted privately by the woman concerned, and although working in conjunction with the midwife they focus on quite separate areas. This is a good example of where a dually qualified acupuncturist/midwife could operate, putting all skills into practice at the same time and thus offering women a choice within the national health service. Since the technology and equipment required for acupuncture analgesia is minimal it could just as easily be taken out into the community for home births as well.

In occupational health

The September 1984 edition of *Occupational Health* describes how acupuncture has successfully been incorporated into a large occupational health service in Scotland and one or two smaller ones in the Midlands and South East.[14] Nurses, in cooperation with medical officers, have used acupuncture in the workplace, finding it a safe, effective and lasting method of treatment. In many cases the time taken to effect a cure is quicker than with conventional methods, often reducing time off work. Here the occupational health nurse can combine both acupuncture treatment and traditional practice in one role.

Further scope

By extending the roles of nurses, the potential scope for the nurse/acupuncturist is extensive. District nurses or health visitors working in the community could use acupuncture where appropriate as well as carrying out their usual tasks. Similarly in hospital out-patient departments, pain clinics and possibly in accident and emergency departments, nurses could combine all their skills to provide more effective patient-oriented treatment. However, given the limitations of the nurse's role and the present organisational structure of the health service, much of this is unrealistic until major changes are made in our current medical system.

The effectiveness of acupuncture in physiotherapy departments has also been widely recognised where it is frequently used not only as a method of pain relief, but also to help extend the range of movements limited by arthritis (and similar conditions), and in some cases to overcome paralysis following strokes.

The importance of thorough training

Although this widespread use of acupuncture is encouraging, there is much to be concerned about the way in which it is practised. First, it is a medical system in its own right and as such requires a thorough training. A knowledge of modern western medicine is no guarantee of an automatic ability to practise acupuncture. Second, and most importantly, there is an implicit danger of any complementary therapy being used in a purely mechanistic symptom-relieving way, and much care must be taken to ensure that the holistic potential of acupuncture is not compromised by inclusion into medical orthodoxy. This is a subject to which I shall return later.

CURRENT RESEARCH

Since orthodox medicine has acquired the dubious status of being 'scientific', all medical research is based on quantitative measurements of efficacy. Anything that is unable to be measured in traditional linear terms of weight, number, time or volume remains outside the realms of medical discourse.[15] Chinese medicine does not work within these parameters (neither, would I suggest, does much of what constitutes orthodox medicine). However, this does not mean that acupuncture is an irrational system of medicine. It is in fact both logical and theoretically consistent based on centuries of empirical observation.[16] But its standards of value are measured in terms of Yin/Yang, the relationship of the microcosm to the macrocosm, and the energetic phases of the Five Elements — qualitative rather than quantitative values.

Since acupuncture's profile in the West has become raised, many attempts have been made to explain the scientific rationale behind it, in a way that is consistent with modern physiology and biochemistry. What has particularly excited western medical researchers is the established connection between acupuncture and the production of neurochemicals within the body. It was found that the application of needles to rats significantly raised their pain thresholds, producing analgesic effects.[17] These chemicals, identified as 'endorphins' are the body's own painkilling substances, produced by many parts of the endocrine system at times of pain, stress or injury. Not only does acupuncture stimulate the production of these chemicals, but it has also been discovered that the process is blocked by administering naloxone, a morphine antagonist. This is certainly the sort of solid scientific evidence that modern medicine is built on, and subsequently the only aspect of acupuncture officially recognised by the medical profession.[18] It is not, however, the whole story. The acupuncture needles must be left in for about 20 minutes before the endorphins reach sufficiently high levels to produce analgesic effects; and yet there are countless cases where immediate pain relief has been obtained within seconds of inserting the needles.

In China itself, acupuncture has undergone comprehensive research and testing over the past 30 years. The results, little known in the West, are quite encouraging and certainly go beyond the present western obsession with acupuncture analgesia and endorphins.

Among the many clinical studies carried out in China between 1958 and 1972 the following are some examples of their findings:

(1) Relating to the digestive system, needling one specific point increased peristalsis in the stomach and accelerated stomach emptying time.[19]

(2) In the circulatory system a certain point was found to increase the leucocyte count in rabbits. However, needling points on rabbits that do not correspond to known acupuncture points produced no visible change in leucocyte count.[20]

(3) In the endocrine system acupuncture could regulate the thyroid gland in cases of endemic goitre. Other examples describe how it increased the secretion of ACTH in the blood of white rats.

(4) In the nervous system, needling certain points can be shown to change the brain ammonia content or affect such things as glucose metabolism in animals.[21]

The fact that biochemical and other physiological changes can be observed as a direct result of acupuncture is obviously good news to all those who believe its efficacy goes beyond mere placebo effect. This clearly demonstrates the body's own self-regulating, self-healing power that can be stimulated by needles rather than immobilised by drugs and surgery. However, it is important to remember that health care is more than just correcting biological malfunctions, whether with acupuncture or drugs. The roots of ill-health lie much deeper than this, and the aim of any medical system should not be just to patch over the faults, symptomatically, but to isolate and expose more fundamental 'causes' leading to education and change both on the social and individual level. New research methods are needed in order to understand what makes us ill in the first place, and to evaluate the efficacy of different kinds of treatment. The inadequacy of 'scientific' double-blind trials has become increasingly apparent, and attempts are now being made to find new paradigms to study 'persons as wholes'.[22]

CONCLUSIONS

The future of acupuncture as an integral system remains highly problematic. There is a fundamental incompatibility between the philosophy of Chinese medicine and that which underlies scientific western medicine. Since science became institutionalised in the West it has been totally dominant and rejects all other forms of knowledge out of hand. A good example of this comes from the recent BMA report on alternative medical systems: 'These systems are incompatible with the corpus of scientific knowledge, and must be rejected by anyone who accepts the general validity of the latter.'[23]

If acupuncture is ever going to be totally accepted it will have to respond to the increasing pressure to explain itself in modern scientific terms. But before this happens serious questions need to be addressed:

(1) What will be the cost if acupuncture is incorporated into medical science?
(2) Are we concerned solely with taking advantage of what is instrumentally useful in Chinese medicine, and not with the reconstruction of its highly coherent system of explanation?
(3) Is the aim to incorporate acupuncture as a technology into the framework of transnational science by providing it with a scientifically rational basis that is completely consistent with physiology and biochemistry, for example, as in the use of acupuncture analgesia?

By regarding acupuncture as effective only as a means of pain relief, the BMA has already successfully reduced it to just another medical technique, totally divorced from its philosophical and theoretical basis. Of course acupuncture should be used to relieve pain wherever possible, but this is only *one* part of a total system that cannot be split up. Without keeping in sight its underlying philosophy, acupuncture will be no more than an assortment of

23

remedies and procedures, and no more holistic than much of orthodox medicine. If we want to gain anything from Chinese medicine, I think it is important not to be put off by unfamiliar Chinese concepts of Yin/Yang, Five Elements etc., but to look beneath this to the spirit of the whole philosophy. This is an acknowledgement of the unity of body, mind and spirit, our inter-action with the environment, and recognition of the whole being more than the sum of its parts.

The future integration of acupuncture into western medicine should not just be based on producing measurable biochemical changes in the body, but more appropriately on trying to understand and learn from traditional Chinese medicine about its general prin-ciples of health. Most importantly, can these confrontations motivate a major re-examination of the fundamental assumptions in western medicine on such basic items as the meaning of health, of disease, the objectives of medical treatment and the relation between medicine and ecology?

Instead of reducing acupuncture to a mechanical technique by compromising it to scientific demands, it is time scientific medicine was challenged to broaden *its* view of health. Of course acupuncture does not have all the answers, nor is it always practised holistically, but it does acknowledge a broader model of health than presently recognised within the medical establishment.

Changes are occurring in the national health service. Take, for example, the growth of the British Holistic Medical Association with its aim to encourage non-drug approaches to treatment and heal-ing.[24] In many hospitals nurse training has become far less task-oriented, while improvements are being made in several medical schools to provide a humane education for medical students.

However, unless the whole system of health care is completely reappraised, these changes will remain at the theoretical level, paying lip-service to the ideal of holistic medicine, but immobilised within a medical system whose existing values fundamentally oppose the spirit of such developments.

NOTES AND REFERENCES

1. For example, the formation of the British Holistic Medical Associa-tion in 1983, a group of doctors and medical students who seek to practise holistic medicine.

2. *Journal of Chinese Medicine*, 9 (April 1982), p. 9.

3. Shanghai College of Traditional Medicine, *Acupuncture: A Comprehensive Text* (Eastland Press, Chicago, 1981), p. 44.

4. *Acupuncture: A Comprehensive Text*, pp. 1–2.

5. *World Health*, the magazine of the World Health Organization (December 1979).

6. R. Croizier, *Traditional Medicine in Modern China* (Harvard University Press, Cambridge, Massachusetts, 1968).

7. *Acupuncture: A Comprehensive Text*, p. 2.

8. *Essentials of Chinese Acupuncture* (Foreign Language Press, Beijing, 1980).

9. F. Mann, *Acupuncture: The Ancient Chinese Art of Healing* (Heinemann Medical, London, 1978), p. 195.

10. *Acupuncture: A Comprehensive Text*, p. 2.

11. *Acupuncture: A Comprehensive Text*, p. 1.

12. R. Dubos, 'Man Adapting to Working Conditions', in *Society, Stress and Disease*, vol. 4 *Working Life*. L. Levi (ed.) (Oxford University Press, Oxford, 1981).

13. For further examples see R.J. Carlson, *The End of Medicine* (John Wiley and Sons, New York, 1975).

14. *Occupational Health* (September 1984), pp. 406–16.

15. See British Medical Association report: *Alternative Therapy: Report of the Board of Science and Education* (1986).

16. T. Kaptchuk, *The Web that Has no Weaver* (Longdon and Weed, New York, 1983).

17. *American Journal of Chinese Medicine*, 2 (1974), p. 203.

18. See the BMA report.

19. *Acupuncture: A Comprehensive Text*, p. 529.

20. *Acupuncture: A Comprehensive Text*, p. 531.

21. *Acupuncture: A Comprehensive Text*, p. 538.

22. J. Heron and P. Reason, 'New Paradigm Research and Holistic Medicine', *British Journal of Holistic Medicine* (April 1984). Also, the recent formation of the Research Council for Complementary Medicine is a positive step towards finding more effective methods of research into complementary medicine.

23. See the BMA report, p. 35.

24. As stated in the aims of the *British Journal of Holistic Medicine* (April 1984).

BIBLIOGRAPHY AND RECOMMENDED READING

Acupuncture: A Comprehensive Text, Shanghai College of Traditional Medicine, (Eastland Press, Chicago, 1981).

Carlson, R.J. *The End of Medicine* (John Wiley and Sons, New York, 1975).

Essentials of Chinese Acupuncture (Foreign Language Press, Beijing, China, 1980).

Kaptchuk, T.J. *The Web that Has no Weaver* (Congdon and Weed, New York, 1983).

Mann, F. *Acupuncture: The Ancient Chinese Art of Healing* (Heinemann Medical, London, 1978).

USEFUL ADDRESSES

International Register of Oriental Medicine
Green Hedges House
Green Hedges Avenue
East Grinstead
Sussex
RH19 1DZ
Telephone: 0342 28567

British Acupuncture Association
34 Alderney Street
London
SW1V 4EW
Telephone: 01 834 3353/1012

Traditional Acupuncture Society
11 Grange Park
Stratford upon Avon
Warwickshire
CV37 6XH
Telephone: 0789 298798

College of Traditional Chinese Acupuncture
Tao House
Queensway
Leamington Spa
Warwickshire
CV31 3LZ
Telephone: 0926 22121

3

Shiatsu

Neil Gulliver

HISTORICAL AND PHILOSOPHICAL BACKGROUND OF SHIATSU

Shiatsu shares its origins with acupuncture and is deeply rooted in the traditions of oriental medicine dating from approximately 5000 years BC. Shiatsu is a form of healing which employs varying degrees of touch from laying-on of hands to firm physical pressure on specific areas or 'points' on the body. Almost analagous to shiatsu is 'acupressure', a widely used term which is often referred to as 'acupuncture without needles'.

Fundamental to shiatsu is the idea that the human organism is totally interrelated with the natural environment with regard to food, water, air, warmth, light, climate, season, etc. Central to this inter-relatedness is the concept of Ki (or Qi, see Chapter 1), a 'vital energy' which is thought to flow through and to animate all life forms. In the human being, Ki is thought to flow in 12 major channels called 'meridians', each relating to a specific organ or physiological function. Along these meridians lie 'points', numbered in order, which are considered to produce therapeutic effects when pressed. For example, the use of 'stomach 25' (Figures 3.4 and 3.6) can often help diarrhoea; and pressure on 'bladder 10' (Figure 3.3) often brings quick relief to headaches. While shiatsu pressure techniques are applied to the surface of the body, it is understood that meridians also flow within the body making connections with internal organs and with each other.

The name shiatsu is a Japanese word meaning 'finger pressure', but its techniques today are far more wide-ranging and can vary from a touch, or laying-on of hands, to deep physical pressure if needed. Mostly shiatsu technique uses moderate physical pressure with much

Figure **3.1:** Stomach meridian (showing right side only) with 'Stomach 25' points 5 cm (2 in.) bilateral to navel

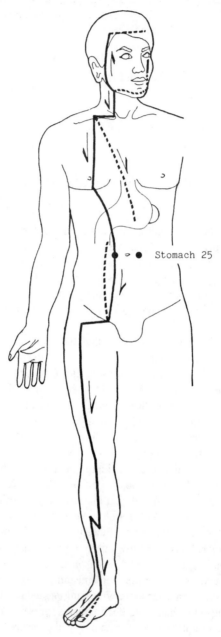

Stomach 25

Figure 3.2: Some points used to treat acute conditions: Bladder 10: between atlas and axis, 2.5 cm (1 in.) bilateral. Small intestine 11: centre of scapula on a level between 4th and 5th thoracic vertebrae. Bladder 25: between 4th and 5th lumbar vertebrae, 4 cm (1 ½ in.) bilateral

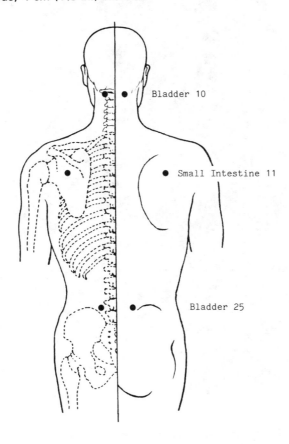

attention to the quality of Ki energy perceived and the tension patterns found in the patient's body. Notwithstanding its long traditional background shiatsu was first developed in Japan specifically as a clinical therapy by Toru Namikoshi who set up his Shiatsu Institute in 1925. By emphasising shiatsu technique in relation to western anatomy and physiology, rather than the oriental concept of meridians and Ki, Namikoshi eventually had his school officially licensed in 1957 by the Japanese ministry of health. Altogether, a combined study of oriental and western medicine appears the best

Figure 3.3: Sitting position (on floor or using upright chair). Pressing bladder 10 to relieve headache and nasal congestion

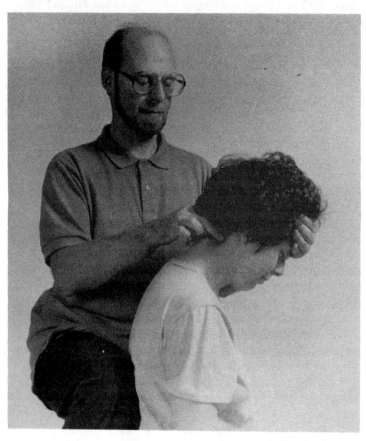

way to ensure the future development of shiatsu. Widely agreed among all schools of shiatsu practice is that the purpose of shiatsu is to activate the body's acknowledged self-healing and self-regulating abilities. In particular, shiatsu derives from two ancient natural healing practices: Do-In and Anma.

Do-In and Anma

Do-In is often described as a form of 'self-shiatsu', whereby specific areas, meridians and points on the body are stimulated by pressure,

Figure 3.4: Lying prone. Pressing bladder 25 to relieve constipation/lumbar pain

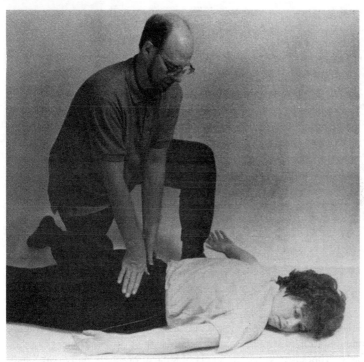

friction, percussion and stretching. Do-In includes breathing techniques and may be considered something like a 'dynamic meditation' in the sense that its aim is to stimulate mental as well as bodily wellbeing.

Anma is the most immediate precursor of shiatsu, and is a technique which has been used in Japan and the Far East for many centuries. Anma is a daily healing/massage practice given in the home for pleasure, relaxation, relief of minor ailments and the prevention of sickness. It involves pressure, kneading and stretching performed according to a general understanding of the meridian system.

YIN AND YANG IN SHIATSU

Vital Ki energy is said to exhibit two opposite but complementary tendencies: the *Yin* tendency is upward and expansive; the *Yang* tendency is downward and contractive. Each meridian is classified as being predominantly more Yin or more Yang, while organs/ meridians are considered to work in pairs: one Yin and the other Yang (see Chapter 2, p. 11, for meridian pairs classified according to Yin and Yang). Simply speaking, this means that in the Yin meridians Ki flows upwards, while in Yang meridians it flows downwards. Meridians run mostly longitudinally along the arms, legs and torso and to all parts of the body. Most of the 12 major meridians begin or end on the fingers and toes. For example, the stomach meridian flows downward to the second toe (see Figure 3.1; and chapter 4 for further discussion regarding Yin and Yang). Total health is said to exist when the flow of Yin and Yang around the body is balanced and equal. When this balance is upset, illness is said to occur.[1]

PRACTISING SHIATSU: WHAT IT INVOLVES

Shiatsu uses non-invasive techniques such as touch, pressure and manipulation to stimulate and harmonise the flow of Ki energy in the body. There are two main levels of shiatsu practice: daily care, and specific therapy.

Daily care

Shiatsu can be very effective in health care when used simply and intuitively (as in the Anma tradition) by the non-specialist. No detailed knowledge of meridians, points or diagnosis is necessary in order to give relaxing and revitalising treatments among friends and family. In hospital a few minutes' daily shiatsu could be given along with everyday nursing care, for example during bed-bathing. Such treatment could be under the direction of an experienced practitioner to ensure maximum effectiveness. This simple level of shiatsu can be useful in relieving such problems as backache, neck and shoulder pain, muscle stiffness, headaches, migraine, stress conditions, constipation, digestive disorders, menstrual difficulties, respiratory problems, depression and general fatigue.

Figure 3.5: Lying on side ('recovery position'). Pressing one of the small intestine 11 points to relieve left shoulder pain/neuralgia

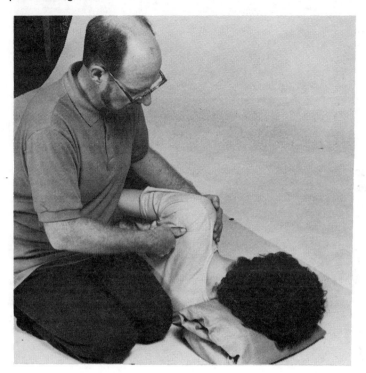

Specific therapy

Full shiatsu treatment by an experienced practitioner will begin with an accurate personal diagnosis based on the taking of a full case history and on the therapist's observation of the patient. In oriental medicine signs such as posture, skin colour, eyes, facial lines, tone of voice, etc. all contribute to the diagnostic picture of the 'whole person', including the patient's general attitude and way of life. As treatment begins the therapist will use touch to confirm and extend the diagnostic picture: feeling for qualities such as tense/flaccid, stiff/loose, hard/soft, hot/cold, dry/wet and developing an overall Yin/Yang perspective of the patient's condition. The shiatsu 'pressure points' (called Tsubo) may be regarded as gateways or valves regulating the flow of Ki into and out of the body and along

33

Figure 3.6: Lying on back. Pressing stomach to relieve diarrhoea/abdominal pain

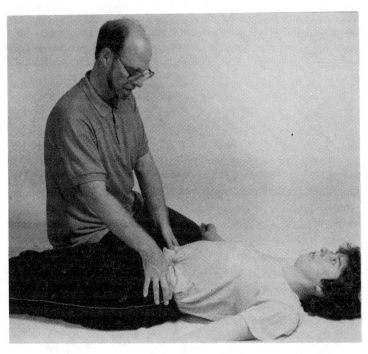

the meridians themselves. The therapist will use superficial and rapid pressure techniques to sedate points and meridians where he finds tension due to an overabundance of Ki. Conversely, he will use deep and holding pressure to tonify those points and meridians that he finds underenergised. Moreover, each meridian/organ is thought to have its positive and negative mental and emotional correlates. For example, if 'liver energy' function is normal then we have patience and humour; if liver is depleted or congested then we tend to be irritable and 'liverish'. It is believed, therefore, that when an individual's Ki forces are properly centred and balanced, self-healing processes become activated at all levels including mental and emotional. Acute conditions can often respond quickly to shiatsu (see Figures 3.1–3.6), while chronic illness may require a course of treatment over several weeks or months. At first, full shiatsu treatment may be given once or twice a week (possibly supplemented by a few minutes' daily care shiatsu) and gradually stepped down to fortnightly or monthly as the patient's self-healing energies are reactivated. Continued 'maintenance therapy' may sometimes be indicated; otherwise it is considered better to help patients towards self-reliance.

RECEIVING SHIATSU

One who receives shiatsu should be lightly but loosely clothed and may be sitting or lying comfortably. Traditionally, shiatsu is always performed at floor level on a suitably padded surface, but a chair or a bed may be used. There are four basic positions for receiving shiatsu: sitting with spine erect (on floor or in an upright chair); lying face down; lying on the left or right side as in the 'recovery position'; and lying on the back (see Figures 3.3, 3.4, 3.5 and 3.6). It is desirable to have a quiet room of sufficient size, ventilated but draught-free, and moderately heated so that the patient is neither too hot or cold. Pillows for extra support may be needed, also a blanket or large towels to cover parts of the body not being worked on. Otherwise no special equipment, clothing or facilities are needed for shiatsu.

GIVING SHIATSU

The shiatsu therapist may wear normal everyday clothing provided it allows for movement and floor-work if necessary. The therapist's condition of health should be good (in other words, better than that of the patient), and normal hygiene standards should be observed particularly with regard to hands, fingernails and hair (long hair should be tied up). Shiatsu is mostly given with the hands, fingers and thumbs, but other parts of the body may also be used to give pressure (for example, arms, elbows, knees and feet).

A full shiatsu treatment usually lasts from 20 to 40 minutes. The therapist will treat specific meridians on all parts of the patient's body: along arms, legs, torso, and especially the spine and the lower abdomen (known as the Hara), selecting certain areas or points for special attention. The hands, feet, neck, shoulders and face are also usually treated in a full shiatsu session. Pressure duration may average 3–5 seconds, but will vary from instantaneous to sometimes holding for half a minute or more. Light touch, stroking, stretching, percussion, friction and hand-healing may also be used. The quality of mutual trust and respect between practitioner and patient is considered especially important.

QUALITY OF SHIATSU TOUCH

This refers to the quality of Ki directed via the practitioner's touch and pressure. In shiatsu tradition, as in martial arts, the Hara (lower abdomen) is held to be the centre of the body's energy and vitality. Posture and all physical action comes from the Hara centre, and the quality of treatment given is thought to be influenced by the therapist's own level of health and consciousness.

In shiatsu practice the giver and receiver are seen as playing complementary roles, and the therapy should be viewed as a single process. Although the giver is more 'active' and the receiver 'passive', both are channelling more Ki, or life-energy, in order to promote a more harmonious state of wellbeing. Consequently, both therapist *and* patient benefit from the shiatsu process. When giving shiatsu correctly, the therapist acts as a 'channel' by which to conduct a better flow of universal Ki energy. In this way it is considered that healing power comes not from but *through* the therapist: from the natural environment at large and hence from the universe. Given with intelligence and due sensitivity it is unlikely that any harmful side-effects will arise from shiatsu.

SHIATSU IN NURSING AND HEALTH CARE: ADVANTAGES AND DISADVANTAGES

It is easy to learn to give basic daily care shiatsu for relaxation, pleasure and the relief of minor ailments. With only a moderate amount of knowledge and experience it is often possible to bring some relief to acute conditions (for examples see Figures 3.1 to 3.6). Selective shiatsu treatments of a few minutes' duration could be given in hospital or home as part of everyday health care, and the use of shiatsu may enrich the relationship between patient and carer to the advantage of both. Practical experience with shiatsu suggests that the element of physical touch in the patient–therapist relationship can help build trust and self-confidence with the patient.

Shiatsu can be used to teach patients simple and enjoyable procedures such as Do-In self-massage to improve his/her own wellbeing, while diagnosis by the observation and touch of an experienced practitioner may reveal early tendencies towards disease which could be avoided with remedial treatment, for example, heart problems or kidney stones. Being economical to the extent that it consumes no technical or material resources, shiatsu can be used almost anywhere at any time. In emergency situations where no medical equipment is to hand, a knowledge of first aid 'pressure points' could be invaluable, such as for revival or to reduce bleeding.

Shiatsu works on a person-to-person basis only, requiring that personal attention and energy is given to patients, and never just routine or impersonal service. Response to shiatsu is sometimes slow, especially with the chronically ill, but its healing effects run deep; time is needed to stabilise a patient's condition. Those health care professionals who give shiatsu must be careful to maintain and develop their own health.

Although shiatsu may seem to have disadvantages in a situation where there is already high pressure of work and shortage of staff, from the patients' point of view, apart from cases where shiatsu is definitely contraindicated (see below), it is difficult to find any real disadvantages in promoting the use of shiatsu in health care.

CONTRAINDICATIONS FOR SHIATSU PRESSURE TECHNIQUES

While an experienced shiatsu practitioner may be able to help in some of the following cases, it is generally advised that those less experienced in shiatsu do not give 'pressure' treatments to patients with:

cancer, AIDS, multiple sclerosis, degenerative diseases;
infectious diseases, infectious skin conditions;
high blood pressure, heart conditions, high fever.

However, in cases where pressure techniques should not be used *directly* on an afflicted part of the body, indirect use of shiatsu may be helpful for:

strains, sprains, dislocations, fractures, broken bones;
arthritis, rheumatism, inflammatory conditions;
burns, rashes, skin conditions;

pregnancy and childbirth (normal and 'abnormal' conditions).

The above lists are not intended to be exhaustive, but indicate the perimeters of shiatsu pressure technique; whereas a gentle healing touch or laying-on of hands may be used for anyone in any condition who will derive comfort and support from the touch of a caring person.

PROBLEMS IN EVALUATING THE EFFECTIVENESS OF SHIATSU

To date, there has been little objective scientific evaluation of shiatsu. However, it may be possible to relate scientific studies conducted on acupuncture, hand-healing or therapeutic touch to shiatsu. The reason for this lack of scientific evaluation is threefold:

(1) Individual practitioners and shiatsu teaching organisations do not have sufficient funding for extensive research projects.
(2) Established medical research foundations — particularly those connected with drug interests — are unlikely to fund research into shiatsu therapy. This may be because of difficulty in establishing an appropriate methodological research approach.
(3) Consequently among shiatsu practitioners there is a general feeling that orthodox medical/scientific research criteria are not yet adequate to evaluate shiatsu.

In his reaction to the British Medical Association's Board of Science and Education report on 'Alternative Therapy' Dr Brian Inglis sums up this feeling on behalf of many 'alternative' practitioners: 'Most of the therapies' organisations stayed away, realising that it was going to be a waste of breath. Some relented, when invited to give evidence, and have regretted it. Those who co-operated have been let down . . .'.[2]

Any worthwhile investigation of shiatsu must make qualitative (subjective) as well as quantitative (objective) evaluations, whereas orthodox science holds to the latter as being the only measure of truth. The objective, distanced, non-involved posture of orthodox scientific enquiry leaves it effectively blind to whatever cannot be measured, timed or weighed. While there may be much useful measurement-based research to be done in shiatsu, its value as far as patients are concerned must lie very much in the subjective and experiential realm. Only patients can say if shiatsu makes them feel better.

Researchers could gain a more comprehensive evaluation of shiatsu by learning some of its techniques and experiencing its effects at the hands of an experienced practitioner. In its holistic sense shiatsu treats people rather than diseases, implying that full research would value individual 'anecdotal' feedback. Serving the holistic approach of shiatsu, traditional theory (involving Ki and Yin/Yang) would be seen as 'qualitative' working concepts rather than quantifiable measures. In order to comprehend such therapies as shiatsu any true research must add experience to knowledge. Perhaps it is time for medical science to discover that it has a heart as well as a head.

SHIATSU TODAY

Shiatsu is still very much a developing healing art, not just an ancient technique which has been resurrected. As a clinical therapy it challenges both eastern and western medical traditions to come together and augment each other. Shiatsu is enjoying a rapid growth of interest and influence in the West, and its teachers in Europe and America find that increasing numbers of students are attending courses as much for the sake of self-development and personal growth as from the desire to pursue professional training.

Significant among those who have made shiatsu known in the West are a number of Japanese teachers who have also written books (see bibliography, p. 40). Probably the most popular and comprehensive beginners' manual is Ohashi's *Do-It-Yourself Shiatsu*. The Do-In books are also very readable for beginners, with well-illustrated practical directives for self-massage and self-healing techniques with reference to certain Tsubos and the meridian system. Namikoshi's approach to shiatsu is more clinical and anatomical, providing a bridge between traditional technique and western medicine and pathology, whereas Yamamoto and Masunaga's work stems from the 'subtle energy'-based concepts involving Ki and Yin/Yang theory. Masunaga, a medical scholar as well as a shiatsu Master, is considered by many to have made a major contribution to shiatsu by extending the meridian system and developing subtle diagnostic techniques further. Always emphasising life and health rather than having an excess preoccupation with pathology, Masunaga wrote that shiatsu treatment '[improves] the patient's life by working from the roots of his existence and enlightening the patient to a better way of life'.[3]

Advantages of Do-In

Learning some Do-In ('self-shiatsu') is highly recommended as a way of studying shiatsu, and is an essential prerequisite for giving it to others. A few minutes' Do-In could help one into a more energetic mood at the beginning of the day. At work, a knowledge of Do-In might help relieve stress, headaches, muscular stiffness, or sharpen judgement and concentration when important decisions have to be made. Do-In is also a very enjoyable way for revitalisation, and perhaps brings a sense of confidence in that it helps one become master of one's own energy. Even at a simple level, shiatsu and Do-In could be used with great enjoyment and benefit in both hospital or home situations.

NOTES AND REFERENCES

1. Readers may note some differences between shiatsu and acupuncture regarding conventions of the Yin/Yang classification. Being a dynamic philosophy of change, Yin/Yang theory often appears paradoxical. The cyclical ebb and flow of Ki implies that, like night and day, each tendency must give rise to its opposite: for example, darkest night (Yin) must eventually give rise to daybreak (Yang). More important than one's initial choice of the Yin/Yang classification, however, is to develop an understanding of how Ki moves and changes.

2. *Journal of Alternative Medicine*, 4 (7) (July 1986), p. 3.

3. W. Masunaga, *Zen Shiatsu* (Japan Publications, New York, 1971), p. 41.

BIBLIOGRAPHY AND RECOMMENDED READING

de Langre, J. *First Book of Do-In*. (Happiness Press, Megalia, California, 1971).

de Langre, J. *Second Book of Do-In*. (Happiness Press, Magalia, California, 1974).

Masunaga, S. *Zen Shiatsu*. (Japan Publications, New York, 1971).

Namikoshi, T. *The Complete Book of Shiatsu Therapy*. (Japan Publications, New York, 1981).

Ohashi, W. *Do-It-Yourself Shiatsu*. (George Allen and Unwin, London, 1976).

Yamamoto, S. *Barefoot Shiatsu*. (Japan Publications, New York, 1979).

Genesis Books, 188 Old Street, London EC1V 9BP (telephone: 01 250 1869) always has a good range of shiatsu and Do-In books in stock. A mail order booklist is available on request.

APPENDIX: COURSES AND INFORMATION ON SHIATSU

The central organisation for shiatsu in the United Kingdom is the Shiatsu Society. Information is available on membership, books, local introductory courses and professional training. A list of registered practitioners and teachers is supplied on request. The Society is run voluntarily and by subscription to provide information on shiatsu. While having no commercial affiliation to any particular school of shiatsu its other main function is to regulate admission to its register.

Please enclose a large s.a.e. with your enquiry to: Elaine Liechti (Secretary), The Shiatsu Society, 19 Langside Park, Kilbarchan, Renfrewshire PA10 2EP, Scotland.

For courses in Suffolk and further information, contact: Neil Gulliver, Lifeways, 2 Capondale Cottages, New Lane, Holbrook, Ipswich, Suffolk IP9 2RD.

4

Macrobiotic Diet

Neil Gulliver

INTRODUCTION

The British diet and state of the nation's health continues to be severely criticised by various authorities including the British Medical Association,[1] the NACNE Report,[2] and the Faculty of Community Medicine at the Royal College of Physicians.[3] Notwithstanding the more positive dietary trends emerging in some other western European countries and in North America, we in Britain remain seemingly addicted to refined sugar, white bread, excessive salt and saturated animal fats.[4]

Since food constantly refuels and rebuilds the body there can be little doubt that the quality of our food affects the quality of our life. This simple connection is being realised by increasing numbers of people who are experimenting in their daily lives with dietary changes which are mostly directed toward wholefoods and a more vegetarian style of nourishment. However, many people find that their pathway to 'the right diet' is obscured by complicated nutritional theories and by food fashions which constantly overturn each other. Against this background the macrobiotic approach to food brings a simple overview to the understanding of human diet. The reason for this connects with the word 'macrobiotic' which requires that we first take an overview or holistic perspective about eating and only then should we focus down on microscopic nutritional details.

Coming from the Greek, *macro* means 'great' and *bios* means 'life'. So to eat 'macrobiotically' means to choose our foods with an awareness of how our own life is supported by the greater natural environment. Eating, like breathing, provides a fundamental biological link with the environment which supplies essential needs such as light, warmth, air, water and food. Macrobiotic eating begins with the simple requirement that what we eat connects with where we are geographically. Consequently a macrobiotic diet involves eating foods which are whole, locally grown and seasonally fresh.

Despite Florence Nightingale's advice long ago regarding fresh locally grown vegetables in promoting patients' health and recovery,[5] diet has only recently become regarded as an important aspect of medical care. Within this context macrobiotics could offer health care not only an enhanced dietary intake but a coherent way of using food more creatively in everyday life both for healing and for general vitality. Improved dietary practice among nurses and health care workers is likely to improve personal effectiveness and ability to cope at work, especially under stress. Eating is an integral part of everyone's daily life, so diet should not be seen as a special food regime or therapy (the word diet comes from the Greek *diaita* meaning 'path of life'.

Perhaps the broadest and most socially valuable application of macrobiotics today is to bring as many people as possible to a higher level of health through better daily eating patterns. There is an urgent need to improve the average British diet, the effects of which can no longer be complacently ignored.[6] Nurses, the medical profession and health care workers can play a key role in personally introducing many individuals to a better level of health through improved dietary practice.

FOUR MACROBIOTIC DIETARY PRINCIPLES

Relationship with environment (or external dietary balance)

Macrobiotic dietary practice makes for balance and harmony between the individual and the environment, emphasising foods that are whole, local and seasonal.

Internal dietary balance

Macrobiotic eating promotes health and harmony within the individual according to the balance of Yin and Yang energies of foods. Yin/Yang theory is discussed below, but see also Chapters 2 and 3. This embraces scientific nutritional concepts such as acid/alkaline or sodium/potassium (Na/K) balance.[7]

Importance of staple foods

A balanced diet consists of staple food plus seasonal and supplementary foods. Staple foods form the main dietary intake; barley, oats, wheat and rye are our traditional staples in western Europe. Every major human civilisation was based on the cultivation of cereals as principal staple food, and for thousands of years grain has been the biological foundation of humanity. For the majority of mankind cereals still remain the principal food, and our expression 'to eat a meal' actually means 'to eat grain'.

Importance of cooking

The skill, understanding and art of the cook is of paramount importance, also the cook's love and care for those who are to receive the food. Macrobiotic cooking involves the conscious application of 'fire' to foods. This is thought to enhance its nutritional and subtle energetic qualities. Furthermore, as human beings, cooking enables us to modify the Yin/Yang balance of foods, giving us greater creative and adaptive freedom than animals.

KI IN FOOD: YIN/YANG BALANCE

Fundamental to macrobiotic thinking on food is the concept of Ki (or Qi, see Chapter 2; there is no equivalent English word), which may be interpreted as 'subtle energy' or 'life force' within food. Ki energy is thought to flow through all living things and to exhibit a blend of two opposing tendencies, referred to as Yin and Yang, which are always seeking balance.

Yin represents the expansive tendency, so Yin foods will be those having a relaxing and dispersive effect on our energy. Conversely, *Yang represents the contractive tendency*, so Yang foods will have a stimulating and concentrating effect on our energy. When our Yin/Yang energies are balanced we are healthy and feel well. Table 4.1 gives some examples of macrobiotic food classification by Yin and Yang.

Table 4.1: Yin and Yang macrobiotic food classification

Extreme Yin
(Very expansive and relaxing; weakening if used in excess)
Alcohol, refined sugar, citrus and tropical fruits, tea and coffee, potatoes and tomatoes.

Moderately Yin
Seasonal local fruits (such as apples, pears, plums)
Seasonal local vegetables (such as carrots, onions, cabbage, turnips)
Dried lentils and beans (such as aduki, chickpeas, blackeye, pinto)

Balanced 'staple' food
Cereal grains are considered the single most balanced food category: for example, barley, wheat, oats, rye, corn, rice, millet, buckwheat.

Moderately Yang
(Animal foods tend to more Yang than vegetable foods)
Fresh white fish, free-range poultry

Extreme Yang
(Very rich, concentrated and contractive; hardening and congestive if used in excess)
Red meat, smoked fish, hard salty cheeses, game, eggs, salt.

Macrobiotic diet, therefore, emphasises 'balanced' and 'moderate' foods around the centre of the Yin/Yang spectrum and advises only very sparing use of the 'extremes'. Western diet, on the other hand, uses plenty of extremes (for example, meat and sugar, eggs and coffee, cheese and tomatoes) with little or no whole cereal staples. Although it is possible to achieve some sort of balance with these extremes, according to macrobiotic thinking the quality of this balance will tend to be erratic, physiologically stressful and conducive to extreme ups and downs of energy and mood. It is believed that a diet centred on whole cereals, beans, lentils, seasonal vegetables and fruit supplemented by fish or fowl (if desired) will create an improved personal Yin/Yang stability and therefore a better all-round balance of health (see the standard macrobiotic diet, p. 49).

YIN AND YANG IN THE BODY

Yang is the tendency to gather, Yin to expand. These tendencies are thought to exist together in all of nature, including ourselves, and describe the movement of vital Ki energies. Within the body, functions such as heartbeat, respiration and peristalsis are all examples of expansion/contraction or Yin/Yang at play as they seek a rhythmic balance. Simple understanding of Yin/Yang can help us regulate our personal balance and day-to-day health, just as reducing salt intake (extreme Yang) will reduce our thirst for liquid (Yin), or moderating meat and egg intake (extreme Yang) may reduce our desire for alcohol, sugar and coffee (extreme Yin). Discovering this simple theory of balance is very exciting because its possibilities in daily life and health care are endless.

HISTORICAL BACKGROUND

Macrobiotics first appeared in Britain during the 1960s due to the teachings of a Japanese writer, healer and philosopher known as George Ohsawa. Originally named Nyoichi Sakurazawa he was born in Japan of Samurai class parents in 1893 but raised to the new western ways of diet and medicine. At 18 he was diagnosed as having advanced intestinal and pulmonary tuberculosis and pronounced terminally ill by western-trained doctors. He began to study oriental medicine and turned to a traditional Japanese diet centred on brown rice and seasonal vegetables. Within a few months he had cured himself of tuberculosis and felt stronger and mentally clearer than ever before. He then determined to devote his life to study, teaching and healing. Over the years Ohsawa developed the philosophy and dietary practice of macrobiotics, drawing upon his oriental traditions and also widely studying western science and thought. George Ohsawa eventually died in his native Japan in 1966, 55 years after being diagnosed terminally ill, after a very active life which had included many years of teaching in the West.

Ohsawa's work was deeply influenced by the writings of Dr Sagen Ishizuka (1851–1910) who advocated traditional 'food-cure' for the prevention and treatment of illness. Ishizuka's food-cure advised a grain-based wholefood diet with special attention to the sodium/potassium (Na/K) balance which he presented as a crucial factor in the recovery and maintenance of health.[8] He classified all illness in terms of sodium/potassium balance and prescribed accordingly. In time Ohsawa came to direct the Food-Cure Society founded in Tokyo after Ishizuka's teachings, and was later to apply the ancient Yin/Yang theory of balance to diet. His counselling methods required individuals to reflect upon why they were sick, advocating that they take responsibility for their own health; he then advised specific changes in diet, attitude and lifestyle.

Figure 4.1: The ancient Taoist symbol suggests the balanced interaction of 'opposites' Yin and Yang) within the 'wholeness' represented by the outer circle

MACROBIOTICS AND THE UNIFYING PRINCIPLE

In 1931, while living in Paris, Ohsawa published *Le Principe Unique* in which he set out his theories concerning food, medicine and his philosophy of the 'unifying principle' (quoted in Ishizuka).[8] The unifying principle holds that everything in the universe is part of an interrelated whole and is one. The ancient Taoist symbol (Figure 4.1) neatly expresses the interplay of opposites within wholeness, asserting them to be of *equal though opposite value* and that one cannot manifest without the other: for example, night and day, spring and autumn, east and west, male and female, Yin and Yang. This symbol also reflects the interdependence of Yin and Yang energies for a harmonious lifestyle. No facets of one's life can be ignored in the unifying or holistic view and each must be considered when moving towards a better balance of health.

Within this context Ohsawa viewed diet as a primary preventive medicine which could also be used to guide emotional and spiritual growth. For optimum health individuals should eat the natural products of their environment in carefully regulated amounts. Ohsawa argued that all sickness related either to an excess of sodium (a Yang element) or potassium (a Yin element), and that health could be restored and maintained primarily by dietary adjustment.[9]

Ohsawa based his teaching of macrobiotics on two principal themes:

(1) *Holistic thinking* as embodied in the unifying principle and involving all aspects of life.
(2) *Macrobiotic dietary practice* as a practical application of the unifying principle towards curing sickness, preventive medicine, and as a basis for personal development and growth of higher levels of human consciousness.

Macrobiotics was proposed by Oshawa as an attitude and a way of life which could be shared by all humanity. Living in harmony

47

with our environment, he suggests, is conducive to personal health and to living in harmony with each other. Although the cultural climate in which it was developed included Taoism, Shintoism, Confucianism and Zen Buddhism, macrobiotics remains non-aligned to any particular religion. It is not a fixed diet nor is it specifically Japanese or eastern. In its more universal and unifying sense macrobiotic dietary principles are attracting growing interest particularly in North America and western Europe. Dr Ishizuka aptly summarised its unifying spirit when he wrote:

> ‘The foundation of the world is the nation,
>   The foundation of the nation is the home,
>   The foundation of the home is the individual,
>   The foundation of the individual is life-spirit,
>   The foundation of life is food.[10]

MACROBIOTIC DIETARY PRACTICE: WHAT IT INVOLVES

> . . . the Sages treated illness first by diet, prescribing a regime of cereal gruel for ten days . . .
>
> Nei Ching Huang Ti
> *Yellow Emperor's Classic of Internal Medicine*
> (China *c.* 500 BC)

Although macrobiotics is not commonly interpreted as a therapy, the results of its dietary application may indeed be beneficial enough to be termed 'therapeutic'. Macrobiotic counsellors and organisations regard their activities as primarily educational. Personal dietary counselling is seen as a one-to-one teaching session which offers clients information and advice which may open up new possibilities of developing their health. If benefit and healing do occur, then it will stem from self-motivation and self-healing.

There are two main levels of macrobiotic dietary practice: standard and specific.

Standard dietary practice is normal everyday eating guided by the four dietary principles and the standard macrobiotic diet shown in Figure 4.2. This level of practice is non-specific in terms of healing and is best used to maintain optimum health. It may also be considered preventive medicine. Experience has nevertheless shown that various minor ailments such as stiffness, muscular pain, headaches, constipation, etc. are often relieved by adjusting toward

Figure 4.2: The standard macrobiotic diet

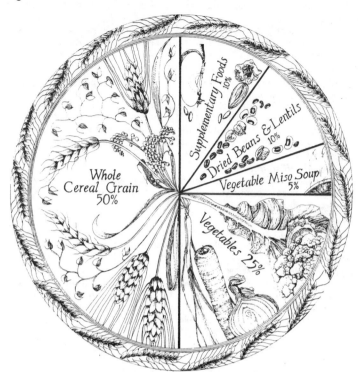

Supplementary Foods 10%

Dried Beans & Lentils 10%

Whole Cereal Grain 50%

Vegetable Miso Soup 5%

Vegetables 25%

this way of eating.

Specific dietary practice is a regime recommended for a given period by an experienced macrobiotic counsellor to alleviate a specific condition. Percentages of the standard macrobiotic diet will be modified and certain foods emphasised or prohibited. Specific dishes, drinks or external treatments may also be advised.

THE STANDARD MACROBIOTIC DIET

The standard macrobiotic diet (abbreviated to SMD) is a guide to both standard and specific dietary practice and is designed to suit the temperate climates of Western Europe and North America. It is offered here on the understanding that the introductory material in this chapter is not intended of itself for direct application. Readers are urged to study the literature and/or seek qualified advice. The

Table 4.2: Percentages for the cooked volume of daily food

Cereal grains (50%)
Barley, wheat, oats, rye, corn, rice, millet, buckwheat, mostly cooked in whole form; some flakes, pasta, bread and flour products for variety.

Vegetables (25%)
Carrot, parsnip, celery, leek, onion, turnip, swede, pumpkin, cauliflower, cabbage, kale, broccoli, cress, radish, cucumber, lettuce, sprouts. A variety of cooking methods may be used to enhance seasonal variety. *Sea vegetables* (for example, dulse, kelp, laver, kombu, wakame, arame, nori[11]) are considered important in macrobiotic eating and are valued for their mineral, iron and iodine content.

Vegetable-miso soup (5%)
Homemade vegetable soup (often including sea vegetables) to which is added miso, a fermented soybean paste thought to be rich in B vitamins including B_{12}.

Dried beans and lentils (10%)
Aduki, mung, chickpeas, haricot, blackeye, split peas and various lentils; often pressure-cooked or casseroled to make protein-rich dishes.

Supplementary foods (10%)
Seasonal fruit, seeds, nuts. Animal foods are selected for freshness and natural quality, being used only in modest amounts (for example, fish, seafoods, free-range fowl, game); fresh white fish is the preferred source of animal protein.

following notes illustrate the scope of the SMD, but fuller food lists can be found in such books as Cowmeadow's *Introduction to Macrobiotics*. The percentages in Figure 4.2 refer to the cooked volume of daily food as it appears in Table 4.2. It is important to remember that the SMD is a guideline only, and that it is capable of great flexibility to suit individual or therapeutic needs.

Staple foods (cereal grains, dried beans and lentils) lend themselves well to storage and transportation, enabling us to eat them all year round and to extend our nutritional horizons. The principle of 'local and seasonal' applies especially to perishable produce, vegetables and fruit. The importation of some Japanese products such as soy sauce, miso and various sea vegetables, is a transitional phase until it becomes economically viable to produce our own equivalents. The application of macrobiotic diet implies the development of regionally based and ecologically sustainable modes of organic agriculture.

Please note that cereal grains *cooked and eaten in their whole form* (such as pot barley, brown rice, millet) do not give rise to excess weight gain *no matter how much is eaten*, whereas *flour products* (such as biscuits, cakes, pasta) may if used excessively.

The standard macrobiotic diet should not be seen as a restrictive regime but as a focus and foundation for healthy eating. If you are in good health and your daily eating is sound then it is important to have the flexibility to enjoy eating out socially with friends or relations, making the best food choices in the circumstances. Food should never become a preoccupation, but a simple grasp of macrobiotic principles may help you to use food in a more positive way to serve health, both personally and professionally.

GUIDELINES FOR TRANSITION TOWARDS STANDARD MACROBIOTIC DIET

Let food be your medicine
Hippocrates ('Father of modern medicine', 460–370 BC)

Any dietary health care programme must begin with at least the following three considerations.

(1) Nurses and health care workers must take a critical but constructive look at their own dietary practice.
(2) They must make or request for more enlightened food choices in hospital menu and staff canteens.
(3) They must support each other to make positive dietary adjustments.

Try to acknowledge the *fundamental importance of food* for the care of self and others, giving appropriate time and thought to food preparation and planning, especially if you work at night or irregular hours. Choose the best quality foods available, organic where possible. Your main food items (cereal grains, vegetables) are fairly cheap, and since the 'standard' diet would not normally include meat, cheese, butter or eggs your weekly food bills will probably be much lower.

Gradually re-equip your kitchen with good quality cookware and utensils (such as cast iron, stainless steel, heavy enamel — *not aluminium*), which may be viewed as a long-term investment both economically and healthwise. Cook with flame (gas) in preference to electricity, since it tends to give you more control and variety in your cooking techniques (top chefs always choose gas!). For

Figure 4.3: Sample day's macrobiotic menu

Sample
Day's Macrobiotic Menu

~ Breakfast ~

Real Oat Porridge with Barley Malt
or Roasted Sesame Seeds
Wholemeal Toast with Pear & Apple Spread
Herb Tea or Bancha Tea

~ Lunch ~

Vegetable -Miso Soup with Watercress
Aduki Bean Casserole with Sauteed Onions
or Fillet of Plaice with Ginger Sauce
Tambouli Salad
(Bulghur Wheat, Vegetables & Dressing)

~ Dinner ~

Creamed Carrot & Barley Soup with croutons
Brown Rice with Chestnuts
Steamed Vegetable Selection
(Parsnip, Cauliflower & Broccoli)
Stir-fried Tofu (Soya Beancurd)
with Parsley Sauce
Apple Fool with Almonds

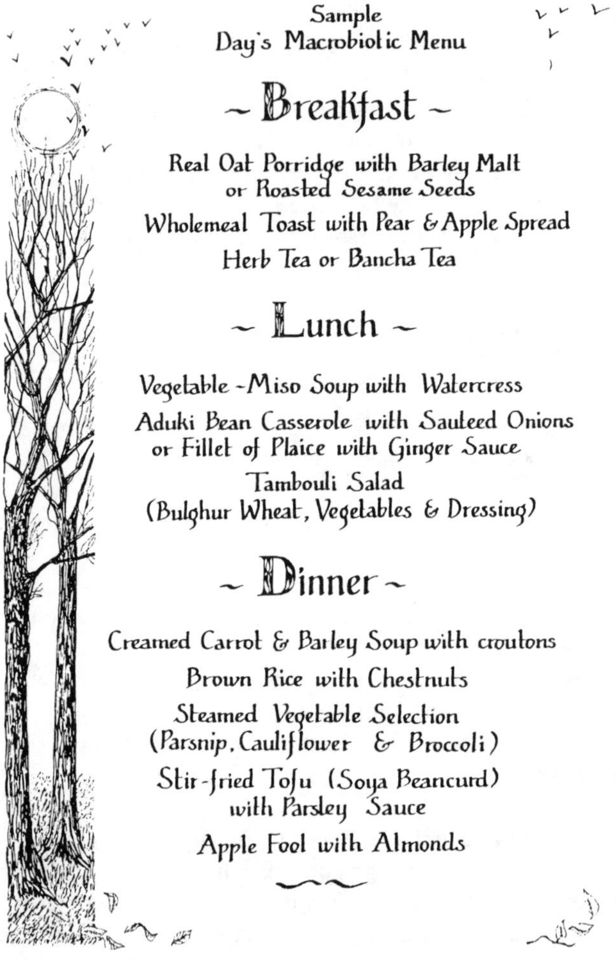

example, it is extremely difficult to cook delicious wholefood macrobiotic dishes using electricity and aluminium cookware. Microwave cooking is *strongly advised against* since it is thought to be destructive to the vital Ki forces within food.

Make a *programmed dietary transition* that feels comfortable but does not lose momentum or sense of purpose. Some aspects can change immediately, such as cutting out refined sugar or coffee. Try to see macrobiotics as enriching your food experience, not restricting it. The standard macrobiotic diet can be the basis for simple daily eating, specific dietary practice in case of illness, or for rich and colourful party catering (Figure 4.3 shows a sample day's menu).

Please remember to chew very well: at least 50 times per mouthful! This applies to everything you eat, but it is especially important when eating moderately seasoned natural foods and the complex carbohydrates derived from root vegetables and cereals in particular. The more thoroughly you chew the better such foods will taste and the more beneficial their effect, as salivary enzymes convert carbohydrates into complex sugars.

Foods to use more

The following foods should be used more or introduced into your diet.

(1) Organic cereal grains, mostly in whole, unrefined form.
(2) Fresh vegetables and fruit, seasonal and geographically local.
(3) Vegetable protein sources, such as dried beans, lentils, tofu.
(4) Fermented soy products, such as soy sauce, miso.
(5) Fresh white fish, such as plaice and sole.
(6) Unrefined 'cold-pressed' vegetable oils, used moderately.
(7) Sea vegetables, such as dulse, kelp, laver, kombu.

Foods to use less

The following foods should be used less or eliminated from your diet.

(1) Refined sugars, including white, brown, syrup, molasses.
(2) Refined carbohydrates, such as white bread and all white flour products.
(3) Saturated animal fats, especially red meats and all dairy fats.
(4) Stimulant beverages, such as 'normal' tea and coffee.
(5) Refined salt, replace with sea salt, used sparingly.
(6) 'Nightshades' and tropical produce, such as potatoes, tomatoes, aubergines, bananas, citrus fruits.

STUDIES OF MACROBIOTIC DIET

Although no large-scale studies have examined the macrobiotic dietary approach there is an increasing amount of anecdotal experience which appears to be supported by scientific knowledge. For example, developments in macrobiotic approaches to cancer are very encouraging.[12] An interim report on Kaposi's sarcoma in relation to AIDS sufferers will hopefully prompt further research.[13] The American research team has reported,

> We have been sequentially studying, since May 1984, the immune function in a group of (19) men with Kaposi's sarcoma who had chosen to forgo conventional medical treatment. They are following a vegetarian (macrobiotic) diet . . . The average calculated lymphocyte number/mm^3 increased from 1122 at diagnosis to 2584 two years later . . . A linear regression analysis model predicts that lymphocyte number becomes normal within this two year period . . ..[14]

Some small-scale studies, also in America, have indicated that those who follow a macrobiotic diet will have lower than average blood pressure, and serum cholesterol levels and be less at risk of serious heart disease.[15]

Macrobiotic organisations would no doubt welcome more scientific research and attention. Unfortunately, they do not have the large research funds available to commercial food and drug companies who for obvious reasons would be unlikely to investigate any possible benefits of a diet based on simple, inexpensive and relatively unprocessed foods.

Healthy daily eating, while certainly requiring more consideration than convenience foods, does not *take* time and energy but *gives* more time and energy to your life. Personal experience has shown that with good food you will need less sleep and so have more time in which to enjoy your extra vitality!

Perhaps the key to using diet as an aid to healing lies in encouraging a sense of gratitude: for food, life, nature, friends and everything that gives us nourishment. Grateful and appreciative patients are often the ones who thrive best. In dietary care *transitional cooking* is a crucial factor: to present appealing dishes that combine something new with something familiar. We may prepare food for others but we cannot chew it for them or digest it or feel grateful on their behalf. However, through food lovingly and consciously prepared, it is often possible to awaken a person's true health and spirit of gratitude.

MACROBIOTIC DIETARY PRACTICE IN HEALTH CARE

A truly good physician first finds out the cause of the illness and having found it, he first tries to cure it by food. Only when food fails does he try medicines.

Sun S'su Mo (China, 581–682 AD)

Macrobiotic dietary practice offers a number of advantages in health care because it is simple, personal and can benefit large numbers of people in many different circumstances. Balanced daily eating is a fairly simple matter using the dietary principles and standard macrobiotic diet to guide our judgement, and a macrobiotic meals service will require the special degree of personal care and attention likely to be of benefit to patients. Also, for reasons mentioned above, food budgets could prove cheaper than for 'normal' eating, even allowing for best/organic quality and the use of some imported products such as miso soybean paste. In hospitals or residential communities large numbers of people could benefit (even unknowingly) from a 'macrobiotically conscious' kitchen.

Orthodox medicine or natural therapies such as shiatsu (see Chapter 3) may be used in cooperation with macrobiotic eating, and appropriate diet could aid recovery from surgery, drugs or radiotherapy.[16]

The whole question of diet and macrobiotic principles may appear unimportant or too much trouble to some health workers and administrators, since more staff and a higher degree of kitchen skills are needed for an effective macrobiotic food programme. Macrobiotics demands a commitment to developing our own health and understanding before we can care more effectively for others.

CONCLUSIONS

The difference between macrobiotic and modern scientific approaches to human nutrition is that science usually seeks only to answer the question, 'What do *I* need?', whereas macrobiotics views nutrition in the wider sense of, 'How can I eat to relate harmoniously with my environment?' Orthodox nutritional science reveals fragments of truth which may be interesting and sometimes useful, but lacks a holistic and unifying view. Macrobiotics, on the other hand, begins from an overview which seeks to understand the orderliness of nature and of our place within it, so that diet is seen as part of a cooperative relationship rather than an egocentric demand upon the environment.

Ultimately, however, there is no conflict between the analytical/scientific and unifying/macrobiotic viewpoints since they tend to complement each other. A varied macrobiotic diet provides all the nutrients required according to analytical science.[17] Hopefully, macrobiotics and nutritional science will increasingly blend together to form a truly comprehensive understanding of human diet which will embrace both the 'great' and the 'small', the macroscopic and the microscopic.

It would seem that nurses, medical staff and health care workers are uniquely placed to encourage healthier ways of eating among large numbers of people at a time when the desire for better dietary understanding is on the upswing. A macrobiotic orientation in this respect would tend to move health care further towards simplicity and self-reliance, and would represent an increased investment in human-based rather than technology-based values.

NOTES AND REFERENCES

1. BMA Board of Science Report: *Diet, Nutrition and Health* (BMA, London, March 1986).

2. The NACNE Report: A Discussion Paper on Proposals for Nutritional Guidelines for Health Education in Britain. (National Advisory Committee on Nutrition Education, London, September, 1985.)

3. Royal College of Physicians: Faculty of Community Medicine report (Royal College of Physicians, London, June 1986).

4. C. Walker and G. Cannon, *The Food Scandal* (Century, London, 1985), part I in particular.

5. F. Nightingale, *Notes on Nursing. What It Is and What It Is Not* (Duckworth, London, 1859. Facsimile Reprint, Harrison and Sons, London, 1970).

6. See BMA, *Diet, Nutrition and Health*, NACNE Report; RCP Report.

7. Preliminary studies of food chemistry in terms of Yin/Yang balance can be found in H. Aihara, *Acid and Alkaline* (George Ohsawa Macrobiotic Foundation, Oroville, California, 1971).

8. S. Ishizuka, *A Chemical Nutritional Theory of Long Life*. Published in Tokyo (1897), this was the original book that influenced Ohsawa. (Reissued Tokyo, 1975, Japanese edition only.)

9. G. Ohsawa, *The Unique Principle* (George Ohsawa Macrobiotic Foundation, Oroville, California, 1931, edited by H. Aihara, 1978). This is a major theme throughout the book.

10. S. Ishizuka, *Shokomotsu Yojoho: Ichimei Kagokuteki Shoku-yo Tai Shin Ron* (Tokyo, 1899).

11. See nutritional information in M. Kushi and S. Blauer, *The Macrobiotic Way* (Avery, Wayne, New Jersey, 1985), p. 53.

12. See anecdotal accounts and scientific references in M. Kushi and A. Jack, *The Cancer Prevention Diet* (Wellingborough, Thorsons, 1984), and A.J. Sattilaro, *Recalled by Life* (Boston, Houghton-Mifflin, 1982).

13. Letter in the *Lancet* (July 1985) entitled 'Patients with Kaposi's Sarcoma Who Opt for No Treatment'.

14. Preliminary report by E.M. Levy, J.C. Beldekas, P.H. Black and L.H. Kushi, 'Patients with Kaposi's Sarcoma Who Opt for Alternative Therapy' (Department of Microbiology, Boston University School of Medicine, Boston, Massachusetts, and Division of Epidemiology, University of Minnesota, Minneapolis, Minnesota, 1986).

15. F. Sachs, A. Donner, W. Castelli, D. Chronomeyer, P. Pletka, H. Margolius, L. Landsberg and E. Kass, 'Effect of ingestion of meat on plasma cholesterol of vegetarians', *Journal of the American Medical Association* (1981), 246, pp. 640–4.

16. Personal account, E. Nussbaum, 'Choosing Life', *Macromuse*, 26 (periodical), Bethesda, Maryland.

17. See nutritional information in Kushi and Blauer, *The Macrobiotic Way*, pp. 4, 47, 48, 51 and 52.

BIBLIOGRAPHY AND RECOMMENDED READING

Aihara, H. *Acid and Alkaline* (George Ohsawa Macrobiotic Foundation, Oroville, California, 1971).

Aihara, H. *Basic Macrobiotics* (Japan Publications, New York, 1985).

Cowmeadow, M. *Macrobiotic Cooking* (Cornish Connection, Penzance, 1986).

Cowmeadow, M. *Macrobiotic Desserts* (Cornish Connection, Penzance, 1986).

Cowmeadow, O. *Introduction to Macrobiotics* (Thorsons, Wellingborough, 1987).

Kotzsch, R.E. *Macrobiotics Yesterday and Today* (Japan Publications, New York, 1985).

Kushi, M. and Blauer, S. *The Macrobiotic Way* (Avery, Wayne, New Jersey, 1985).

Kushi, M. and Jack, A. *The Cancer Prevention Diet* (Thorsons, Wellingborough, 1984).

Ohsawa, G. (1931) ed. Aihara, H. *The Unique Principle* (George Ohsawa Macrobiotic Foundation, Oroville, California, 1978).

Ohsawa, G. ed. Aihara, H. *Macrobiotics: An Invitation to Health and Happiness* (George Ohsawa Macrobiotic Foundation, Oroville, California, 1971).

BOOKS AND COURSES

Macrobiotics and its dietary practice are usually taught via:

(1) Personal health counselling for an individual or family.
(2) Public lectures and classes, including practical cooking.
(3) In-depth courses and training programmes in macrobiotic cooking, dietary counselling, shiatsu and healing.
(4) Books, magazines and periodicals.

The principal stockist of macrobiotic books and publications in the United Kingdom is: Genesis Books, 188 Old Street, London EC1V 9BP (telephone: 01 250 1868). A mail order booklist is available on request.

The main macrobiotic teaching centre is in London and there are a number of regional centres offering classes and dietary counselling services. Contacts and information from: Jon Sandifer, The Community Health Foundation, 188 Old Street, London EC1V 9BP (telephone: 01 251 4076). The Foundation offers dietary counselling and is the parent organisation for the East West Centre (public clases) and the Kushi Institute (extended courses).

USEFUL ADDRESSES

Northern Ireland
Gerry Thompson
Macrobiotic Natural Living Centre
48 Fitzroy Avenue
Belfast
BT7 1HX
Telephone: 0232 238 318.
Republic of Ireland
Patrick Duggan and Anne Currie
'Teac ban'
6 Parnell Road
Harolds Cross
Dublin 6
Telephone: 0001 783 943.

5

Reflex Zone Therapy

Hazel Goodwin

INTRODUCTION

A few years ago not many people had heard of reflex zone therapy, or reflexology as it is more commonly called; but recently there has been a great surge of interest in the complementary therapies and I no longer encounter blank looks when I say I am a reflex therapist or that I teach reflexology.

In spite of the tremendous advances in medical science over the past century, people are realising that orthodox medicine does not have all the answers, and not all medical professionals have the right approach to health.

'Holistic health', as defined by the British Holistic Medical Association, is an approach to health that emphasises the health care of the whole person, not only on the physical, but also on the emotional, psychological and spiritual levels.[1] It recognises every individual's capacity for self-healing and accepts that disease is often the result of stress, faulty habits, destructive thought patterns and unfavourable social conditions. Patients are expected to take a responsible, active part in any treatment programme which may include orthodox medical care and remedies, psychotherapy and instruction in self-help skills.

Many of the students on my reflexology courses are nurses and health care workers who are seeking additional ways of helping their patients. A knowledge of reflexology is an ideal adjunct to the skills of anyone working in the caring services, and health care workers are in a particularly good position to practise reflex zone therapy, or to direct patients towards a therapist, where they feel it could be of benefit.

One of the greatest benefits of reflex therapy is in the reduction of stress within the body. Now no one can deny that nurses and health care workers are engaged in a stressful occupation, and I find it very interesting to see how the students on my courses respond to working with each other during the sessions. Over the weeks, after giving and receiving regular practice treatments, most of those taking part feel positive benefits: they are calmer, healthier, have greater energy and a more optimistic outlook on life. I know of many ex-students who continue to give each other reflexology treatments as an 'insurance' against illness and a way of helping them to cope with the stresses of their work.

Reflex therapy, besides being a therapy in its own right, is ideally suited for use in collaboration with orthodox medicine and nursing care or with other complementary therapies. It is a safe, non-invasive treatment, cooperating with the body's own healing processes to induce a state of balance and wellbeing. It also often helps the body to counteract the side-effects of drugs and is very valuable in aiding recovery after illness, operations or fractures.

WHAT IS REFLEX ZONE THERAPY?

'Reflex' in the context of reflexology means the 'reflection' of all the organs, systems and structures of the body onto the feet or the hands. Reflex therapy is the practice of working on these reflexes in such a way as to produce a relaxation and response in the corresponding body regions. By applying controlled pressure with the thumbs or index fingers to the reflex points and areas on the feet, the body is stimulated to achieve its own state of equilibrium and good health. Pressure on the reflexes not only affects the organ or region of the body but also influences the relationship between different functions, processes and parts. Although it is possible to work on the hands or feet, the foot reflexes are more sensitive and it is generally more efficacious to work with them.

ZONE THEORY

Reflexology is based on an ancient Chinese concept that every part of the body is connected by energy pathways which terminate in the feet, hands and head. These energies pass through zones in the body, but do not cross the spinal column as do nerve pathways. Zone theory is a system of organising the body into ten longitudinal zones

Figure 5.1: The Ten Zones

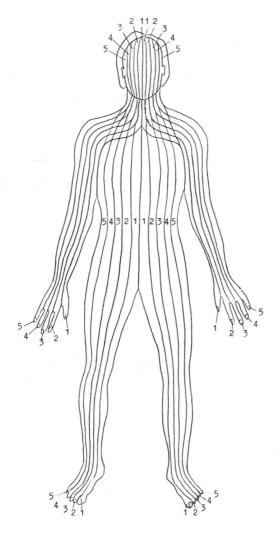

from the toes to the top of the head and down the arms to the fingers (Figure 5.1). Any tension, congestion or dysfunction in any part of a zone will affect the whole zone. Therefore, pressure applied to any part of the zone, but particularly to the terminal reflexes, will cause a reaction throughout that zone.

The position of the reflex areas on the feet correspond closely to

Figure 5.2: Medical correspondences

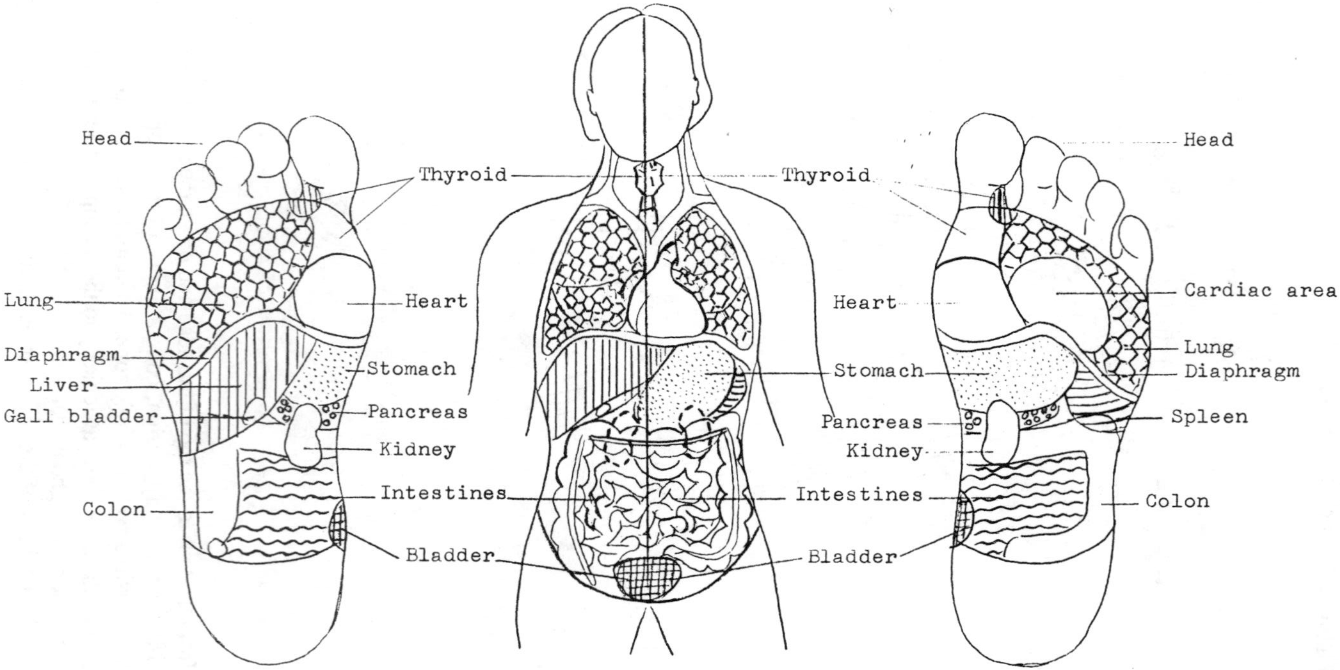

Figure 5.3a: Skeletal reflexes.

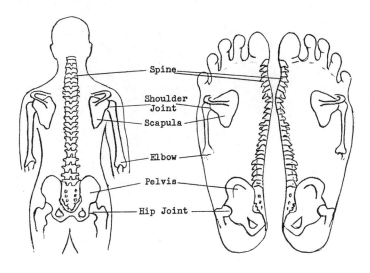

Figure 5.3b: Skeletal reflexes

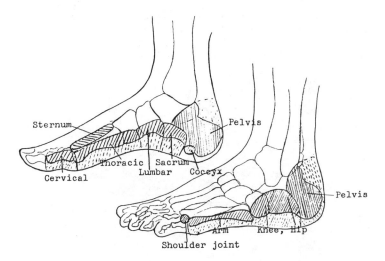

Figure 5.4: Reflexes on dorsum

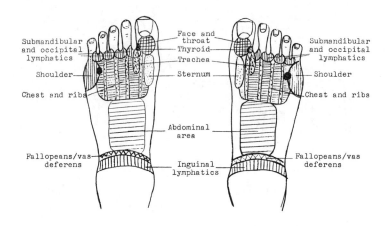

Figure 5.5: Reflexes on the sides of the feet

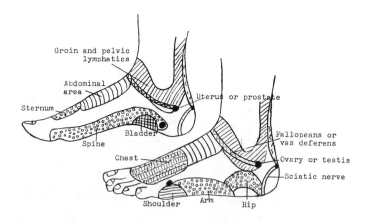

Figure 5.6: Lateral divisions

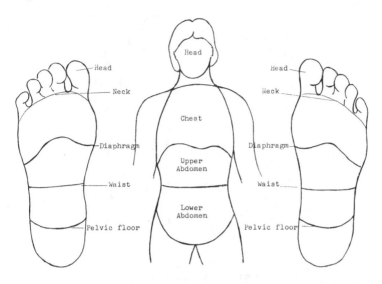

the relative position of the organs, glands or structures of the body itself and are located in the same zone — each foot representing half the body (Figures 5.2, 5.3a and b). As both the feet and the body are three-dimensional, so reflex areas are found not only on the soles but also on the dorsum and sides of the feet and ankles (Figures 5.4 and 5.5). The feet can also be divided laterally to correspond to areas of the body. The divisions are drawn at the neck, the diaphragm, the waist and the pelvic floor (Figure 5.6).

As we are working on the whole person, not just the physical body, these lateral divisions can also correspond to other levels of being: the head reflexes to the intellect and thinking; the chest to the emotions and feelings; the upper abdomen to action — the way one operates in the world, work situations or occupations; the lower abdomen to relationships — the ability to give and take, to flow and adapt; while the heel area corresponds to movement and transformation, physical, mental and spiritual. It is interesting that in ancient Chinese philosophy these divisions also correspond to the five elements: ether, air, fire, water and earth (Figure 5.7).

Figure 5.7: Philosophical correspondences

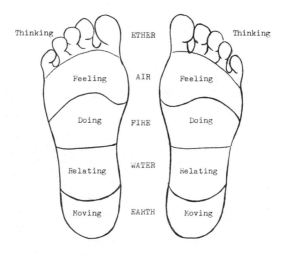

THE HISTORY OF REFLEX ZONE THERAPY

Treatment of the body by using pressure points on the feet is not new. It was used in China and India over 5000 years ago, and a wall painting in the ancient Egyptian tomb illustrates its usage there in 2,300 BC[2] (Figure 5.8). A number of American Indian tribes have also used for many centuries very similar methods for treating disease and relieving pain.[3]

Whether folk medicine in the West ever used such methods is not recorded, though in the 16th century a number of European doctors published papers describing ways of treating internal organs through the use of pressure points.[4] The Italian sculptor, Benvenuto Cellini, is also said to have used pressure on his hands and feet to relieve pain.[5] However, it was not until the end of the 19th century that zone therapy was rediscovered and introduced to the western world by an American ear, nose and throat specialist, Dr William Fitzgerald. His main interest was in the use of pressure points on the hands, and to a lesser extent on the feet, to relieve pain and induce anaesthesia in specific areas and enable him to perform minor surgery on his patients without anaesthetics. He used a variety of mechanical devices for stimulating the points including rubber bands and metal combs; and on a number of occasions he publicly demonstrated the effects on his colleagues by pressing points and then sticking pins into the anaesthetised parts![6]

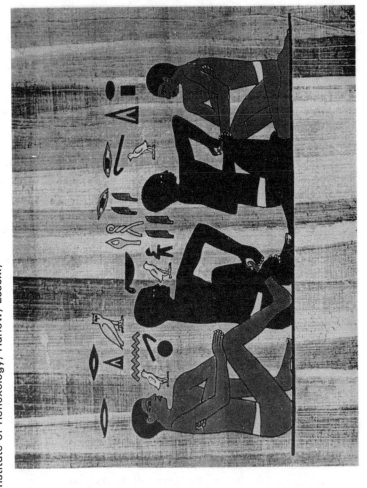

Figure 5.8: Detail from wall painting in physician's tomb, Egypt 2330 BC. (Reproduced by permission of the International Institute of Reflexology, Harlow, Essex.)

In 1917 Dr Fitzgerald and Dr Edwin Bowers jointly published a book describing their methods,[7] which showed diagrams of the ten zones and presented a rough 'map' of the internal organs on the soles of the feet. They also coined the term 'reflexology' for the study of the reflexes. In 1919 Dr Joseph Shelby Riley published a book called *Zone Therapy Simplified* in which he introduced his discovery of the horizontal zones of the feet.[8] Since then many books have been written, a great deal of research has been carried out, and a number of people have made important contributions to the development and acceptability of reflex therapy.[9]

The study of reflexology as taught by the International Institute of Reflexology is based on the work of Eunice Ingham Stopfel, an American masseuse who studied and worked with Dr Shelby Riley. She spent many years painstakingly locating the reflexes on the feet, compiling charts and evolving her own method of 'compression massage'. In her book *Stories the Feet Can Tell* published in 1938, Eunice Ingham describes her methods and experiences with reflexology; this, and its sequel *Stories the Feet Have Told*,[10] probably brought reflexology to the public notice more than anything else.

Because of the developing, dynamic nature of the therapy, the student will find some diversity between the different schools both in the exact location of some of the reflexes and the method of treatment. I do not think this is important. What is important is to learn the principles properly, to practise regularly and to be open to the new insights, deeper understanding and the personal growth which inevitably comes to those who practise any therapy with sincerity.

THE STRUCTURE OF THE FEET

When studying reflexology it is useful to have some idea of the structure of the feet, for this not only helps to locate the pressure points corresponding to the various glands and organs, but also gives an understanding of the function and importance of the feet themselves.

The foot is a beautiful and complex piece of structural engineering, designed for bearing the weight of the body and transporting it over the ground. There are 26 bones in the foot (Figure 5.9). These bones are held together by 107 tough fibrous ligaments which limit the movement of the bones but allow an impressive degree of flexibility. The body's weight is transmitted by the tibia to the talus and distributed to the heel and the metatarsals. When standing, the heels

Figure 5.9: Bones of the feet

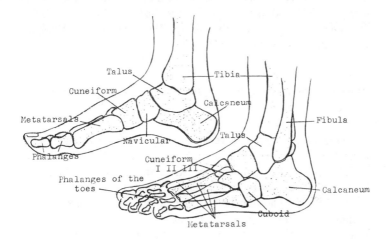

and the heads of the metatarsals support most of the weight; the bones are locked together with the ligaments under tension thus forming a solid arch which is supremely efficient for supporting weight. When walking or running, weight is released from the arches, the bones unlock and the foot becomes a flexible, active spring which absorbs shock and adapts to uneven ground. In fact the feet are healthiest when walking barefoot over rough ground. Wearing shoes and walking on pavements inhibits the natural strengthening movement of the bones, ligaments, tendons and muscles; and long periods of standing weaken the ligaments, flattening and lengthening the arches of the feet.

THE FEET AS SENSORY ORGANS

Not only do our feet support us and carry us around but they are important sense organs conveying vital information to the brain. There are 7200 nerve endings in each foot connected by way of nerve pathways, which loop through internal organs to the central nervous system. All coordinated movement depends on how the body perceives and interprets its internal and external environment. The more accurate the sense perceptions, the better able the body will be to achieve balance and harmony in every aspect of living.

69

Primitive man walked barefoot and the soles of his feet were massaged and stimulated by contact with the ground, nerve endings were activated and messages relayed to the brain. We are in danger of losing much of the sensitivity of the feet through lack of stimulation to the sensory nerve endings.

STIMULATING SENSORY RESPONSES THROUGH REFLEX THERAPY

Working on the feet with reflex therapy helps to re-establish the close contact between the feet and the whole body, and between the body and the environment by stimulating nerve endings and providing a deep sensory experience.

As we get older the body's functioning is influenced by the accumulated experiences of a lifetime. Both the mind and the body store memories of past illnesses, physical hurts, emotional pain, and psychological and social stresses. We shift weight to relieve pain in joints or organs, tense some muscle fibres to ease others, droop our shoulders when unhappy, tighten our stomachs, clench our jaws, find excuses, become anxious, or otherwise modify the way we use our minds and bodies. These modifications become habitual and affect our posture, functioning and thinking. Much of the body's 'wear and tear', often attributed to ageing, is due to the way we misuse ourselves.

Reflex therapy can help in reprogramming the mind and body by sending signals through the feet to encourage the body to reassess and rebalance its internal environment, in much the same way that when walking barefoot over the ground the feet send messages to the brain enabling the body to assess its position in space and so allow balance and movement to take place.

HOW DOES REFLEX ZONE THERAPY WORK?

There is plenty of empirical evidence that reflex therapy works and that by pressing points on the feet specific parts of the body are affected.[10] I know from personal experience that this is so, and many books written about reflexology contain a section on 'case histories', based on the patients' records which are kept by all reputable therapists. But just how and why reflexology works is not so clear.

Zone theory explains it in terms of energy channels, like meridians in acupuncture, connecting every part of the body. Eunice Ingham postulated that the malfunctioning of any organ, gland or part of the body causes crystalline deposits of uric acid and calcium to form on nerve endings in the feet. These crystals slow down circulation and lymph drainage and impair muscular activity in the corresponding part. Compression massage, she claims, breaks down these crystals which are then reabsorbed and eliminated so promoting improved circulation throughout the body.[11]

Other theories include the hypotheses that reflex points are nerve receptors;[12] or that muscles store repressed psychological tensions and inhibitions that are released when reflex points are pressed;[13] that reflex therapy works directly on the lymphatic system;[14] or that treatment releases lactic acid residues.[15] No doubt there are others but none really explains how such a detailed mapping of the body onto the feet takes place.

Reflexology is not the only therapy or system that uses a projection of the whole body onto a part. Iridology, as a diagnostic technique, uses the iris of the eye as an image of the internal organs (see Chapter 14); in palmistry the character, life events, and health are mapped onto the palms of the hands; oriental diagnosis projects the body onto the face, and auriculotherapy onto the ear, while Ampuku is a method of treating the body through corresponding reflexes on the abdomen. But how or why an image of the body is projected onto a part has not, as far as I know, been explained.

Perhaps it can be understood as working in a similar way to the hologram, a three-dimensional picture produced by laser beams which fix a coded image onto a two-dimensional photographic plate. One unusual attribute of a hologram is that if the plate is broken any fragment can be used to reconstruct the whole image, which means that all the information about the whole picture is contained in every part. It could be that systems which use reflections or pictures of the whole body projected onto a part are based on the concept that every part of the body, indeed every cell, contains a complete image and understanding of the whole; and that such therapies and diagnostic techniques are utilising the body's ability for self-perception and self-knowledge.

THE PRACTICE OF REFLEX THERAPY

Reflex therapy is not a mechanical procedure but an intimate attunement between two people with the aim of promoting positive good health on all levels. Both are involved in the process and it is important for the therapist to have the right attitudes. The practitioner has skills which should be used with compassion and dexterity but without emotional involvement or concern about the outcome of the treatment. The object is not to take away pain or disease but to use the hands in such a way that energy is always flowing outwards; for all healing is self-healing, and the therapist's aim is to act as a catalyst for the patient's own healing energies, not to take responsibility for his/her health.

Both the hands and feet are extremely perceptive sensory organs capable of transmitting and receiving accurate and subtle messages. If the therapist is tense or anxious, with unruly thoughts or emotions, this will be transmitted to the patient causing reciprocal tension and unease. So it is important, before starting, to be calm and centred. Then, with hands relaxed and open, gentle contact is made with the feet. The first touch is important and sets the tone for the whole treatment.

Touching people in a caring way is an important aspect for any therapy and, as the hands and feet are particularly sensitive, a special kind of communication is established when practising reflex therapy. I always feel, when working on the feet, that I am 'tuning in' not only with my client's energies but also with a higher, organising, interconnecting life force which is beyond the range of our normal perceptions but which contributes to healing and homeostasis on all levels.

Before beginning a treatment both the patient and the therapist should be comfortable and relaxed, breathing quietly and deeply from the diaphragm, the patient's arms uncrossed. Ideally the feet should be level with the therapist's chest, the patient sitting or reclining, with back and knees well supported, in such a way that eye contact can be maintained throughout.

The feet should first be explored with the hands, maybe with eyes closed, to tune in and pick up signals. There are a number of relaxing techniques that can be used to release tension from the feet, the body and the mind (Figures 5.10 and 5.11). These include light stroking, rotating the ankles, moving the toe joints, and massaging gently with fingers, thumbs or knuckles, easing out tension wherever it is felt. These preliminaries, although not part of the actual treatment, can be used very beneficially by anyone to help partners, friends or patients to relax and feel better. Try holding and caressing someone's feet, letting your hands move intuitively,

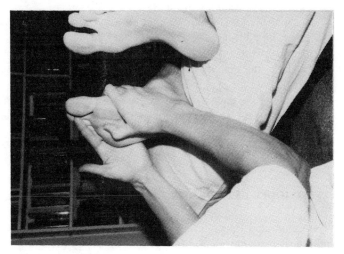

Figure 5.11: Thumb 'walking' over the lung area

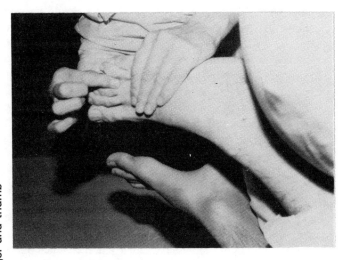

Figure 5.10: Pressing with the Eustachion Reflex with finger and thumb

feeling the flow and exchange of energy which is so much a part of the healing process for both the people involved.

It is not the aim of this chapter to teach reflex therapy but to introduce the subject to the reader. It is an exact and intricate science best learned from a qualified teacher. Training as a reflex therapist also includes the study of anatomy and physiology which is essential for anyone wishing to practise professionally. So only a brief description of the methods used is given here, but hopefully enough to encourage further interest. Details of the different schools, courses and seminars can be obtained from the professional bodies listed at the end of this chapter (p. 83).

TECHNIQUES USED IN REFLEXOLOGY

The thumb and finger technique used in reflexology is unlike any other massage movement. Work is done mostly by the thumb which, by moving only the distal joint, crawls like a caterpillar in a forwards direction over the reflex areas in a specific sequence. Needless to say, the nails must be kept short to avoid digging into the feet. Treatment usually starts on the toes, or head area, then proceeds over the sole, round the ankles, and finally, using fingers in the same 'caterpillar walk', the dorsal aspect of the foot is covered (Figure 5.12). Thumb and finger movements should be slow and rhythmic and the pressure even. Reflex points to the glands and organs are pressed by a 'hook-in and back-up' technique which accurately pinpoints the reflex (Figure 5.13). Points can be tender and people's sensitivity varies, but usually any pain felt is quickly dispersed with treatment. Any very tender places may need a little extra attention as this can mean a blockage or depletion of energy in that area. The aim is to stimulate healing and bring relief, not to inflict pain, so pressure should always be adjusted to the feet being 'worked'.

During treatment the foot should be held in such a way as to give a sense of comfort and security. Both hands remain in contact with the foot throughout, providing leverage and support. Most schools advocate starting on the right foot and working over that foot before moving to the left, although this is not always the case. There is a great proliferation of schools, particularly in the United States, and they all have their own individual variations. However, it is universally accepted that, as reflex therapy is aimed at helping to restore health and balance to the whole person on all levels and not just

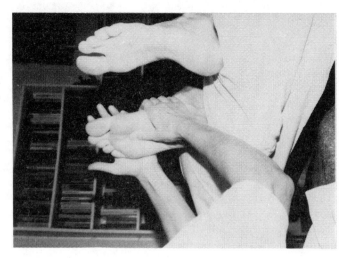

Figure 5.13: Pressing the solar plexus reflex

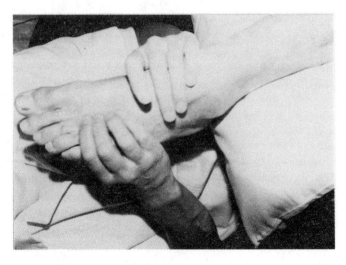

Figure 5.12: Finger 'walking' over the chest area

relieving symptoms, the whole of both feet must be worked in every treatment although emphasis can be given to symptomatic or causal areas.

A treatment usually lasts for between a half and one hour and, if possible, the patient should rest for a while after the session. Occasionally there is a temporary reaction as the body rids itself of released toxins. This will not last long and should be seen as part of the healing process. If there is a reaction the patient should be advised to eat lightly and drink plenty of liquids.

CONDITIONS HELPED BY REFLEX THERAPY

The main benefits of reflex therapy are relaxation and the normalisation of the body's functions. A great many of today's diseases and disorders are the result of stress which causes disruptions to the normal functioning of the body. By inducing a state of relaxation, muscular and emotional tension is released, circulation improved, blood supply to vital organs increased and the elimination of toxins and waste matter is hastened. Treatment encourages the body's internal communication systems to work more efficiently; this is particularly helpful if there is any hormonal imbalance, especially during menopause or in cases of dysmenorrhoea.

There is, indeed, a wide range of conditions which can be helped by reflex therapy: stress-related problems such as allergies, asthma, insomnia, depression, anxiety, migraine and so on; disorders due to muscular tension, back pain, fibrositis, neck and shoulder problems; and it can also be of great benefit in restoring balance to the endocrine and autonomic nervous system.

However, as mentioned earlier, it is not an alternative to, nor a replacement for, other forms of treatment, and a therapist will always refer patients to doctors or other health care therapists for treatment or examination if at all necessary. Reflex therapy works well in conjunction with other medical remedies and is a great aid to recovery.

CONTRAINDICATIONS IN REFLEX THERAPY

Although reflex therapy is a safe and effective way of aiding the body to restore health and balance, there are some conditions when it is not appropriate. It should not be used when a person has an

acute infectious disease or febrile condition, or if there is inflammation of the lymphatic or venous systems. It is also not advisable to
give treatments during unstable pregnancies or when there is deep
vein thrombosis, and in cases of severe cardiac disorders it is as well
to obtain advice from the patient's doctor before giving therapy.

Children can be treated with reflex therapy and usually love it,
but pressure must be very light and the session short. Old or frail
patients also need light, gentle handling, and babies' feet should only
be held, caressed and lightly stroked.

If the foot itself has corns, calluses, bruises, sores or fungal infections those areas should be avoided. And if it is not possible to work
on the foot at all because of injury, verrucas, infectious skin
diseases, oedema, etc., then reflex therapy should be given on the
hands.

HAND REFLEX THERAPY

The structure of the hand is similar to that of the foot and the location
of the reflexes corresponds closely although they are nearer together
on the hand (Figure 5.14). There are some situations when it is
easier to work on the hands than on the feet and the technique and
procedure is the same. Even if it is not perhaps quite as efficacious
as foot reflex therapy, it is nevertheless a very beneficial and
pleasurable experience.

The easiest position is for the therapist to sit facing the patient so
that the hand can rest on the knee. Holding and caressing the hand
is a natural way to bring comfort to another person and any hand
massage, given with compassion, will help the patient to relax and
release tension.

REFERRAL AREAS AND CROSS REFLEXES

At the beginning of this chapter it was noted that reflexology is based
on the zonal system and the relationship between all parts of the
body lying within the same zone. Referral areas are parts of the body
that relate to each other through the zones — the thumb is in the
same zone as the big toe, for instance, and the eye is in the same
zone as the kidney.

Cross reflexes work on the theory that some parts of the body
reflect others — the arm is a reflection of the leg, the wrist of

Figure 5.14: Hand reflexes

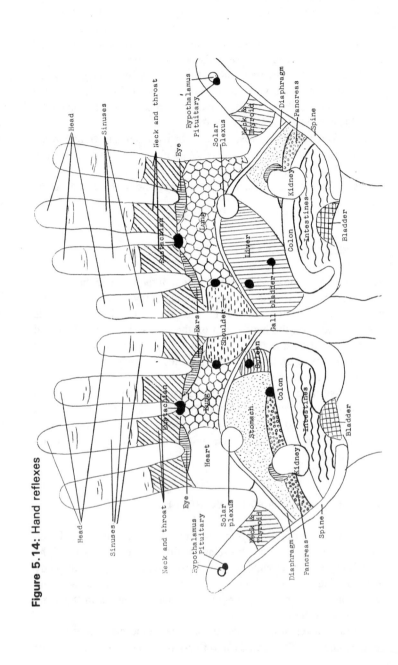

Figure 5.15: Cross-reflexes

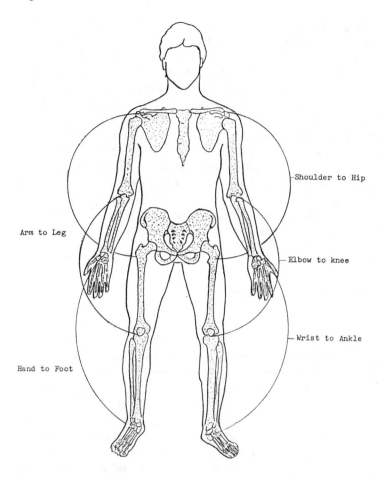

Shoulder to Hip

Arm to Leg

Elbow to knee

Wrist to Ankle

Hand to Foot

the ankle and the hip of the shoulder, etc. (Figure 5.15).

These principles of zones and cross-reflexes can be used to relieve pain and promote healing in parts of the body that cannot be touched directly because of injury or inflammation. For instance, an injury to the knee will cause tenderness not only to the knee reflex on the foot but also in the referral area of the elbow located in the same zone. Working over referral areas with thumbs or fingers, and using holding pressure on tender points, will help to direct healing energy to the injured part. These areas can also be used in self-healing.

79

SELF-TREATMENT

It is perfectly easy to give oneself a hand or foot reflex therapy treatment or to relieve pain in injured parts by using referral areas and cross-reflexes. The main disadvantage in treating oneself is that it is not possible to obtain the deep relaxation that comes when receiving a treatment from someone else. Also the stimulus to the healing process is not as strong because one's energy is operating on a closed circuit. However, there are nevertheless great benefits to be obtained from self-treatment. Sensory signals are transmitted from the reflexes to the corresponding body areas increasing self-perception and evaluation, and mobilising the healing process; circulation is improved with all the advantages that it entails; nerve pathways are cleared, and the foot or hand is made more flexible and receptive. Also, since our hands and feet are always with us it is possible to fit in short treatments while for instance, watching television, travelling or taking a bath.

PROFESSIONAL STATUS

Unlike any other country in the western world, common law in England permits the practice of any therapy or treatment which has not been specifically proscribed, provided, of course, that the practitioner does not contravene any other civil or criminal laws. This is an important freedom and is less open to abuse than is sometimes claimed. After all, a practitioner who is no good is not likely to get many clients, and the public is protected from misrepresentation or negligence under existing legislation. However, therapists who work with patients and who wish to be responsible co-workers with the medical profession should be properly trained, maintain a high standard of ethical conduct and also work consciously on their own health and development on all levels.

There is a growing impetus from within the complementary health movement towards forming associations, improving and standardising training and establishing professional status for practitioners.[16]

In 1984 the Association of Reflexologists was founded with the aim of maintaining a high standard of practice among reflexologists, encouraging research, furthering the work of practitioners and providing information to the public. Membership is limited to those with approved qualifications but it is not affiliated to any particular school. Further information and lists of practitioners will be sent on request.

CONCLUSIONS

Reflex zone therapy is based on the following theses:

(1) that pathways of energy flow through zones in the body terminating in the feet, hands and head;
(2) that a 'map' of the whole body is reflected onto the feet and hands, and reflex points connect directly with internal glands, organs and structures;
(3) that working on the feet with compression massage techniques relaxes tension, directs energy and assists the body to achieve its own health potential and homeostasis.

Many people who come to me for treatment have chronic conditions that orthodox medicine has been unable to help. Their doctors have told them that, apart from drugs to relieve the symptoms, there is no cure for their arthritis, or hardened arteries, multiple sclerosis, or persistent backache, and so on. Reflex therapy is not a miracle cure, and not everyone is helped, but treatment *is* based on the premise that given the right circumstances every cell in the body will work together to promote total health and balance.

Reflexology could be a valuable additional skill in the hands of nurses and health care workers. The extra training required could be beneficial since their contact with patients frequently puts them in a good position to practise hand or foot reflex therapy which would augment other forms of treatment. Also, exchanging reflex therapy sessions with colleagues, friends or family would reduce stress, improve relationships and increase the level of health and wellbeing.

I have found that some patients make remarkable progress, especially those who are prepared to accept responsibility for their own health. By doing so they are taking the first big step towards creating the right conditions for self-healing. Obviously, disorders that are the result of years of bad habits, poor posture and wrong diet, for instance, will not be remedied by a few reflexology treatments, although often much relief is obtained. However, reflex therapy does help the body to reassess its own internal environment. Cells are constantly being replaced within the body and by enlisting the body's innate healing powers, sickly cells can be replaced by healthy ones and a process of regeneration and rejuvenation can take place.

Seeking and cooperating with treatment is another step towards health; but it is also necessary for the patient to examine those attitudes, habits and conditions which contributed to the disorder in the first place, and to correct them with proper diet, exercise, posture and positive thinking.

There is a growing interest in holistic medicine throughout the world, and an increasing awareness that our emphasis must be to promote positive health on all levels rather than to cure disease. I look forward to the day when doctors, nurses, complementary therapists, healers, social workers, dietitians and psychotherapists all work together in the health centres of the future to provide a comprehensive holistic health care service for everyone.

NOTES AND REFERENCES

1. From a pamphlet 'What Is Holistic Medicine', published by the British Holistic Medical Association, 179 Gloucester Place, London NW1 6DX.

2. Early 6th dynasty (about 2300 BC) wall painting in tomb of Akhamor (highest official after king) at Saqqara, known as the physician's tomb. The translation reads 'Don't hurt me'. The practitioner's reply is 'I shall act so you praise me'. Reproduced by permission of the International Institute of Reflexology.

3. H. Marquardt, *Reflex Zone Therapy of the Feet: A Textbook for Therapists* (Thorsons, Wellingborough, 1983), pp. 17–19.

4. Marquardt, *Reflex Zone Therapy of the Feet*.

5. Marquardt, *Reflex Zone Therapy of the Feet*.

6. See D. Berkson, *The Foot Book — Healing the Body through Reflexology* (Barnes and Noble Books, New York, 1977), p. 11; K. and B. Kunz, *The Complete Guide to Foot Reflexology* (Thorsons, Wellingborough, 1984), p. 3; and D.C. Byers, *Better Health with Foot Reflexology* (Ingham Publishing Inc., St Petersburg, Flora, 1983), pp. 3–4.

7. W. Fitzgerald and E. Bowers, *Zone Therapy or Relieving Pain at Home*, cited in Berkson, *The Foot Book*.

8. See Marquardt, *Reflex Zone Therapy of the Feet*; Berkson, *The Foot Book*; and Byers, *Better Health with Foot Reflexology*.

9. See Berkson, *The Foot Book*; and Kunz and Kunz, *The Complete Guide to Foot Reflexology*.

10. See D.E. Bayly, *Reflexology Today: The Stimulation of the Body's Healing Forces through Foot Massage* (Thorsons, Wellingborough, 1978, reprinted 1984); E.D. Ingham, *Stories the Feet Can Tell* (Ingham Publishing Inc., St Petersburg, Florida, 1938) and *Stories the Feet Have Told* (Ingham

Publishing Inc., St Petersburg, Florida, 1984); and A. Kaye and D.C. Matchan, *Reflexology Techniques of Foot Massage for Health and Fitness* (Thorsons, Wellingborough, 1979, reprinted, 1984), p. 121.

11. See Ingham, *Stories the Feet Can Tell* and *Stories the Feet Have Told*.

12. See Berkson, *The Foot Book*.

13. See Berkson, *The Foot Book*.

14. See Berkson, *The Foot Book*.

15. See Berkson, *The Foot Book*.

16. Council for Complementary and Alternative Medicine; British Holistic Medical Association; British Association for Holistic Health; Institute for Complementary Medicine; Association of Reflexologists.

BIBLIOGRAPHY AND RECOMMENDED READING

Bayly, D.E. *Reflexology Today: The Stimulation of the Body's Healing Forces Through Foot Massage* (Thorsons, Wellingborough, 1978, reprinted 1984).

Berkson, D. *The Foot Book: Healing the Body Through Reflexology* (Barnes and Noble Books, New York, 1977).

Byers, D.C. *Better Health with Foot Reflexology* (Ingham Publishing Inc., St Petersburg, Florida, 1983).

Ingham, E.D. *Stories the Feet Can Tell* (Ingham Publishing Inc., St Petersburg, Florida, 1938).

Ingham, E.D. *Stories the Feet Have Told* (Ingham Publishing Inc., St Petersburg, Florida, 1984).

Kaye, A. and Matchan, D.C. *Reflexology: Techniques of Foot Massage for Health and Fitness* (Thorsons, Wellingborough, 1979, reprinted 1984).

Kunz, K. and Kunz, B. *The Complete Guide to Foot Reflexology* (Thorsons, Wellingborough, 1984).

Marquardt, H. *Reflex Zone Therapy of the Feet: A Textbook for Therapists* (Thorsons, Wellingborough, 1983).

USEFUL ADDRESSES

Association of Reflexologists
Hon. Secretary
27 Chesterton Road
London
W10 5LY

International Institute of Reflexology
PO Box 34
Harlow
Essex
CM17 0LT

British Association for Holistic Health
179 Gloucester Place
London
NW1 6DX

6

Applied Kinesiology (Touch for Health)

Brian Butler

INTRODUCTION

Applied kinesiology is a method of using a series of muscle tests to locate functional imbalances in the body. It offers detailed, safe, yet highly effective techniques to determine specific ways in which the health of an individual may be enhanced.

Since its discovery in 1964, it has developed into a complex science, due to clinical research undertaken by many chiropractic doctors in the United States. The International College of Applied Kinesiology insists upon very high standards for its graduates. All testing and correction techniques are subjected to rigorous scrutiny and clinical trial. Only those procedures that are reproducible by all properly trained kinesiologists are accepted into the body of information known as 'applied kinesiology'.[1]

BASIC PRINCIPLES OF APPLIED KINESIOLOGY

The basic principles of applied kinesiology may be learned by lay people and interested professionals by studying *Touch for Health*.[2] This simplified synthesis enables anyone to obtain a thorough grasp of the basics of muscle testing in a few evenings or weekend classes. The techniques learned can be applied in effective and practical ways by professional health workers and can also be taught to patients under their care.

APPLIED KINESIOLOGY: A WHOLE PERSON APPROACH

Applied kinesiology may be used to analyse the whole person. Four specific aspects of human function are addressed.

(1) The psychological/emotional conditions affecting the health picture.
(2) Dietary and chemical factors.
(3) Structural considerations.
(4) Energy imbalances.

THE PSYCHOLOGICAL/EMOTIONAL EFFECT ON MUSCLE RESPONSE

It is commonly held that psychological and emotional factors influence greatly the onset, duration and recovery of disease processes.[3] Shock, disappointments, arguments, depression can all have immediate and potentially lasting distorting effects upon the energy of the body, and upon its ability to function at its best. This effect may be demonstrated by testing the way the body can alter a muscle's ability to contract normally when tested.

The gentle caring provided by utilising the simple method of emotional stress relief offered by 'touch for health' has great potential for all dealing with the sick to reduce stress or anxiety simply and efficiently. It offers health care practitioners an excellent tool to enable the patient to deal with stress on any level.

Applied kinesiology can also be used with highly beneficial results to reduce stress and tension experienced by health care staff when caring for others.

DIETARY AND CHEMICAL CONSIDERATIONS

The effect of diet upon health is particularly important. Food can act either in a creative and supportive role where needed nutrients are being ingested and absorbed by the body, or conversely, many people eat foods which actually impede life-giving energy.

It has been shown in DHSS Allergy Clinics that not all organic foods are suited to all people.[4] Wheat, milk, and other common foods cause the highest incidence of allergic reaction. Diet should be tailored to suit the individual. There are foods that, for some people, take more energy than they give to the body. This is apparent in cases where someone has an allergy, but rather less obvious when the food is just not nourishing the person. Here muscle testing may be used to discover the hidden detrimental effects. This is particularly valuable in dealing with hyperactive children.[5]

DRUGS AND CHEMICALS

Virtually all drugs have undesirable side-effects.[6] This does not mean they should not be used, merely that their use should be prescribed as conservatively as possible. The widespread use of antibiotics for minor health problems is causing havoc in the intestinal flora of the nation, with rather unfortunate results.[7] When it is necessary to use these potent killers of bacteria, then post-medicative care for the ensuing bowel imbalances caused by mass destruction of the natural flora could save a fortune in antidepressants and a mountain of human misery.

We are enmeshed in the largest uncontrolled experiment in human nutrition ever conducted. More chemicals, preservatives, colourings, and additives are being used by the food industry in the preparation of foods than ever before. The long-term effects of this upon our own health and that of our children cannot be estimated. It is certainly advisable to avoid all manufactured foods, and give greater emphasis to fish, vegetables and grains that we prepare ourselves. Unhappily though, these too are rarely completely untainted by the effects of sprays and fertilisers.

STRUCTURAL INTEGRITY

The care of the human frame must include regular exercise of the cardiovascular system, carefully avoiding accidental damage. Many people who work hard all day and get very tired think that they get sufficient exercise. This is not always true. For exercise really to be of value the heart rate needs to be increased to no more than twice its normal resting rate,[8] or to whatever a doctor advises in the case of anyone who is really unfit. Failure to get advice upon the most appropriate exercise regime accounts for many deaths each year.

It appears that if one takes regular exercise three or four times a week, which produces the desired increase in heart rate, some deep breathing and some healthy sweat, the chances of dying from a heart attack are greatly reduced.[9]

Applied kinesiology helps greatly in restoring postural integrity in those who have muscular tension. As the imbalances are corrected, posture is improved and a sense of ease and grace returns to body movements.

ENERGY AND LIFE FORCE

In the orthodox approach to training in western medicine, the existence of the life energy pathways known to acupuncturists of the orient for 5000 years is not considered. Happily the medical profession[10] has shown increasing interest over the last few years in the concepts and practice of acupuncture as witnessed by the formation of The British Holistic Medical Association (BHMA) and the Research Council for Complementary Medicine (RCCM).

Knowledge about the electromagnetic energy flows in the body greatly improves our ability to help the sick, especially when this knowledge is used in conjunction with other modalities. When the life force energies are balanced the individual, whether patient or nurse, feels the beneficial effect immediately, and a sense of well-being is experienced even though the person may be unwell or in pain.

WHAT KINESIOLOGY OFFERS

Basic applied kinesiology has a great deal to offer all branches of health care for several reasons. For example, it utilises more natural methods that do not involve the use of expensive equipment, reduces the need for drugs and surgery, and speeds recovery. The basics, learned in a few weekends, can be used with complete safety, and without conflicting in any way with conventional methods of safety.

Applied kinesiology is directed towards individualised patient care incorporating emotional, physical and dietary requirements. It enables practitioners and health care workers to determine each person's specific imbalances that are present at any time, and rectification of these imbalances can lead to an enhancement of the general state of health and wellbeing. In the long term, muscle testing and balancing is directed towards preventing illness, and stabilising the innate healing resources of the body to sustain an optimum level of health.

During applied kinesiological muscle testing, the tester is relieved of the responsibility of attempting to 'diagnose', for muscle testing does not seek to find or attempt to cure pathological conditions. The information derived from patients is not a matter of opinion, but is a reflection of the person's own body response to the questions posed to the body by muscle testing.

HISTORICAL BACKGROUND

The evolution of applied kinesiology is a mixture of chiropractice and osteopathy. The antecedents of today's highly trained practitioners were in some cases 'bonesetters' or natural manipulators with no formal training or qualification.

Applied kinesiology draws these and more disciplines together, such as oriental medicine to provide a systematic method of analysing and treating a very wide range of conditions.

Its origins are found in the research of Dr George Goodheart, DC, a chiropractor from Michigan who examined a patient experiencing severe muscle spasm.[1] One of the muscles tested was the fascia lata, which runs down the outside of the leg from the hip to just below the knee. Goodheart massaged the path of the muscle, and noted that the pain diminished dramatically. He retested the fascia lata muscle to find that its response to being tested was much stronger than before.

Encouraged by this finding Dr Goodheart recalled research undertaken by an osteopath called Chapman at the turn of the century, on reflexes which he had demonstrated improved the flow of lymph.[11] This Goodheart believed was important, since he contended that the efficient circulation of lymph around the body feeds and cleans the intercellular spaces, and is vital to efficient function, and to the maintenance of health and the prevention of illness.

Chapman's reflexes

In studying Chapman's work, it was noted that one of the reflexes followed the path of the fascia lata, and Goodheart discovered that this reflex lay over the muscle it affected. He continued to research the phenomena, and was able to link up points discovered by

Chapman with the muscles and muscle groups to which they related.

These have subsequently become known as the neurolymphatic reflexes of applied kinesiology, a new science born out of the perseverance of Dr Goodheart. The term neurolymphatic reflex was used to explain the immediate effect they have when activated. Weak muscles become strong within a few seconds when these points are massaged if inhibition of the lymphatic flow is part or all of the cause for their weakness.

Bennet's reflexes

Goodheart's research also correlated the reflexes discovered by Bennet. These demonstrated a link with improved blood circulation and muscular strengthening. Bennet had discovered that the circulation of the various organs could be enhanced by touching certain points on the skull lightly. He used a fluoroscope for his research which unfortunately emitted harmful radiation, and possibly hastened his death.[12]

Studying Bennet's reflexes in relation to muscles led to some more interesting connections being made in body circuitry. Now some of the relationships between the musculature and the organs which share a common energy pathway became clearer. Some of these pathways may be understood in relation to the orthodox approach to physiology, others cannot.

THE LINK BETWEEN ACUPUNCTURE AND APPLIED KINESIOLOGY

A connection was made between the ancient oriental concepts of life force or Qi and the pathways of energy called meridians. Meridians have points along their length where needles are applied in traditional acupuncture and were understood to be related to the internal organs. Applied kinesiology has made excellent progress in dealing with hitherto intractable cases because of the insight into body function afforded by integrating the concepts of acupuncture with the fruits of western research.

THE PHILOSOPHY OF APPLIED KINESIOLOGY

The fundamental philosophy of applied kinesiology is that each person has an innate awareness about his/her real state of health.

Applied kinesiology also promotes the approach that health problems and difficulties are a result of improper use of the body. It maintains that health problems stem from the effects of unresolved stress, whether in the psychological or physical realm, or from inappropriate dietary intake. Each person is responsible for maintaining his/her own health. When we abrogate this responsibility, sickness, ill-health or terminal disease results. Unfortunately, the effects of abuse are not always immediately apparent, and may not cause symptoms for many years, so many people frequently assume that being asymptomatic means all is well.

Those serving others as professionals in health care need to have effective ways to keep themselves healthy. They need special protection from the rigours of the stresses and strain involved with tending the sick. Doctors, nurses, dentists, and physiotherapists have to have strong reserves in the bank of health.

In previous generations, most sickness could be accounted for by lack of proper hygiene, poor economic and social conditions. Today, the diseases which maim and kill are more often diseases of degeneration — arthritis, arteriosclerosis, heart failure, and so on. Western medicine frequently concentrates on 'symptomatic cure', after the problem is diagnosed. Applied kinesiology promotes the prevention of illness and self-help by linking closely to the preventive concepts of energy balancing as proposed by the ancient art of acupuncture.

RESEARCH INTO APPLIED KINESIOLOGY

Although the credit for the initial discovery of applied kinesiology in 1964 goes to Dr Goodheart, since then thousands of chiropractors, medical doctors, osteopaths and physical therapists have conducted research on the wider application of applied kinesiology in relation to their own training and professional skills. This has resulted in a remarkable explosion in understanding of human function in a relatively short period, although little has yet been written apart from Dr Goodheart's research papers, and Stoner's work.[12]

Those who have been willing to accept the possibility that muscles may be restored to optimum function rapidly when the cause of weakness has been determined, have entered a new era of greater success in their work.

Orthodox medical doctors and nurses receive such an intensive training for so many years that it is frequently very difficult for them to entertain the possibility that there is an entirely different philosophical way of looking at anatomy and physiology other than the reductionistic perspective taught in medical schools. Those skilled practitioners who have ventured to learn more about complementary therapy and taken weekend courses, have been able to integrate the benefits of applied kinesiology into their practice.

The author of this chapter certainly advocates that basic applied kinesiology should form part of the foundation training of all branches of health care. It offers the advantage of being a simple, reliable method of obtaining valuable information about an individual's state of health and mind by assessing muscle response and then working towards restoring the body's balance.

Applied kinesiology advocates that the recuperative powers of the body work better when the energies of the body are balanced. This is also advocated by other alternative therapies, such as acupuncture and magnetic therapy. Using the simplified methods taught in 'touch for health' classes,* everyone can help themselves and those they care about, and consequently promote a better state of balance.

APPLIED KINESIOLOGY IN HEALTH CARE

The fitter health professionals are, the more confidence they will imbue in those they tend. This will enhance the quality of health care and result in the sick getting well faster. Caring for others involves considerable responsibility to ensure the maintenance of a healthy balanced body and mind. If we do not show a good example, we will not inspire others.

There is currently a crisis of confidence in the medical profession concerning the ability of orthodox medicine to care for patients. The lack of time given to patients has resulted in a regrettable loss of faith in the orthodox approach, to the great detriment of the average man or woman in the street. Also many people are becoming disillusioned

---

* Touch for Health Courses; Brian H. Butler, BA, Touch for Health Faculty Member for Great Britain (see p. 98).

with the continued use of drugs that apparently have no beneficial effect.

The placebo effect is now mocked and derided by many. Do we really care if the person gets well because of a little love and attention, or because of a sugared pill? The important point is that the person could consult someone in whom he/she has confidence to help solve the problem. One possible solution to restoring the confidence of the public in orthodox medicine is for the profession to show its willingness to change in the face of public opinion,[13] to embrace ideas and methods that address a number of minor problems plaguing our society which are not disease as such, but conditions.

For example, conditions of the musculoskeletal frame which give rise to discomfort and pain can be relieved with applied kinesiology rather than with drugs that may produce side-effects. However, a shift in perspective is still required before more orthodox health care practitioners suggest osteopathy, chiropractice, therapeutic massage, or applied kinesiology to their patients.

MUSCLE TESTING

The most important and fundamental tool of applied kinesiology is the method of muscle testing. It forms the basis of the diagnostic assessment of each individual. It is important to understand that this process does not actually diagnose pathological conditions, although a skilled practitioner trained in pathology may obtain indications which would lead him/her to employ this in conjunction with other testing methods to determine whether or not some disease process was present.[14]

Muscle testing checks the unique health pattern of each individual. Professionals may use up to 50 or more muscle tests to make an in-depth assessment. In the simplified approach of the 'touch for health' balance, often just 14 or 15 muscles are tested, one for each main meridian, and those found not to respond fully are corrected. The subject usually notices an immediate change in his/her state of wellbeing.

This is an ideal therapy for busy people involved with the care of the sick. The touch for health balance only takes 3–5 minutes, and can provide an energy boost without taking too much time from the job at hand. For example, one can test the suprinatus muscle by having the patient extend the arm in front and to the side about 45°, and pressing gently on the wrist, then strengthen it by touching the forehead. All this may be accomplished in just a minute or two, and its effect will often help the patient feel a lot better.

This is not called a treatment, because touch for health balances are done routinely as a preventive health care measure much as one might do daily exercises, yoga, aerobics, weight training or jogging to keep in trim. A touch for health balance reaches the parts not corrected by exercise of any kind.

Many different functions such as muscle balance, nutritional deficiencies, and emotional reactions to stress may be checked using standard kinesiological muscle testing procedures, and the areas of balance and imbalance recorded. Wherever there are any inhibiting factors, a change in normal muscle response will be noted. The muscle fibres will not be able to 'fire' their cell bundles strongly or evenly which impedes efficient function.

It has now been established that each organ has muscles that are closely related to it, in that they share the same energy pathways.[1] This has led to the realisation that when muscle function is facilitated, the related organ also benefits since the energy released flows into the circuits common to both. This is why the subject may feel a tangible benefit immediately.

Life force energy controls many functions that are distinctly separate. Applied kinesiology approaches this energy form by assessing a group of five factors at the area of the intervertebral foramen, where nerve fibres branch out from the spinal cord to the tissues and the organs. These five factors are: (1) nerve; (2) lymphatic; (3) vascular; (4) acupuncture meridian; (5) cerebrospinal fluid. Each of these is an energy rather than an anatomical locus, which when correctly balanced conducts energy in the right format to sustain optimum function in the part of the body served by it.

An example may be taken at any level of the spine, for example the junction between the 7th and 8th thoracic vertebrae. At this level, there is believed to be a link with the spleen and the pancreas, and muscles like the latissimus dorsi, middle and lower trapezius, and triceps. Nutritional balance for this circuit may be achieved with the use of foods or tablets containing vitamin B.

ADVANTAGES AND DISADVANTAGES OF APPLIED KINESIOLOGY

Advantages

The main advantages of applied kinesiology as a therapy is that it enables the therapist to determine any needs specific to the individual at any particular time, and to rectify any imbalances. We need to pay more attention to prolonging our healthy lifespan in any way we can.[15]

If a structural imbalance is the primary cause of a problem, then although herbalism or acupuncture or other forms of treatment might help it is possible that the fastest improvement might be achieved by a chiropractor or osteopath.

Conversely, if the problem stems from energy blockages, and meridian imbalances, then the services of an acupuncturist may well be the best first step. However, a striking advantage of applied kinesiology is that it is eclectic in approach, drawing as it does from concepts of acupuncture, osteopathy, chiropractice, herbalism, and numerous other disciplines to provide a more complete system of analysis and treatment than is possible from utilising a single approach. Muscle testing is used to determine which type of treatment would be the most appropriate and effective for this person at this time.

Disadvantages

The principal disadvantages lie in the fact that the patient being tested may be highly sceptical about the validity of the testing. Of course, as in any other sphere, the results must depend upon the professional testing skill of the practitioner or lay person. Testing is frequently referred to as subjective (and therefore by inference, unscientific) by those who consider the scientific process to be the be-all and end-all for evaluating any information. Evaluating muscle testing by conventional scientific methods is rather difficult as many of the factors that influence the testing are extremely difficult to measure.

If someone has many imbalances unresolved over a long period of time, when the next trauma arrives there may be insufficient resilience left to handle the new stressor without some obvious form of disease becoming apparent. This may take the form of mental distress or nervous breakdown, physical pain or discomfort, or biochemical disease, or a combination of all of these. The body heals faster when notice is taken of the main priorities.

CONCLUSIONS

Applied kinesiology is a quick, simple and direct way to assess an individual's state of health. Using touch points, acupuncture energy may be balanced without the need for needles, and blood supply renewed to muscle groups and related organs merely by making contact with the correct location. Lymphatic flow may be dramatically improved, and muscles reactivated by the use of firm pressure on the appropriate reflexes. The improvement in wellbeing in just a few minutes can be quite remarkable.

Using just a few simple tests, invaluable guidance may be obtained about an individual's dietary needs. Foods or other substances which may be causing stress to the body can be quickly discovered. Similarly foods needed to strengthen the muscle groups that are currently inhibited due to insufficient nourishment of a particular kind can be identified. Different muscles and parts of the body need different nutrient emphasis for optimum function.

Many of these simple methods could be employed by nurses trained in muscle testing. It would give them more hands-on contact nursing which is both satisfying and rewarding.

There is no question of the value for those in the nursing profession, subject as they are to physical stresses and strains involved with lifting patients; back trouble is one of the main reasons for nurses leaving the profession. A simple balance of 14 main muscles could well prevent a strain or worse. Dealing with the mental stresses of disease, and all the related human misery, is hard on nurses too, and emotional stress release techniques are of enormous value to the staff as well as the patient.

Applied kinesiology is a new science, so a healthy scepticism for it is a good safeguard. However, rejecting new ideas out of hand because they do not fit with our experience has a very limiting effect upon the growth of individuals and society.

When the author was at school, Everest had not been climbed, the four-minute mile was thought to be beyond the scope of human capacity, and we used to say that there was as much chance of such and such happening as for a man to fly to the moon!

Since then, many have stood upon Everest's summit, the record for the mile is well below four minutes, and many astronauts have since been to the moon.

Applied kinesiological concepts may seem as outrageous to the trained professional as those 'impossibilities' to us 40 years ago. Do not wait, this valuable information is available for you to test and try now. Make it work for you, and for those under your care.

REFERENCES

1. Walther, D.S. *Applied Kinesiology*, vol. 1 Ch. 1 (Systems DC, Pueblo, Colorado, 1981).

2. Thie, J.F. and Marks, M. *Touch for Health* (DeVorss and Co., Marina del Rey, California, 1973) (revised 1979).

3. Pelletier, K.R. *Mind as Healer Mind as Slayer* (Dell Publishing, New York, 1977).

4. Egger, J. *et al.*, 'Diet and Migraine', *Lancet* (October, 1983).

5. Egger, J., Carter, C.M., Graham, P.J., Gumley, D. and Soothill, J.F. 'Controlled Trial of Ologoantigenic Treatment in the Hyperkinetic Syndrome', *Lancet* (9 March 1985), pp. 540–5.

6. Weitz, M. *Health Shock* (David and Charles, Newton Abbott, 1980).

7. Medawar, C. *Social Audit The Wrong Kind of Medicine* (Consumer Association, London, 1984).

8. Walker, M. and Angelo, F. *Rebounding Aerobics* (Edmunds, Washington).

9. White, J.R. *Jump for Joy* (Goldfield Books, San Diego, California, 1981).

10. Forbes, A. *Try Being Healthy* (Whitstable Litho, Whitstable, Kent, 1976).

11. Owens, C. *An Endocrine Interpretation of Chapman's Reflexes* (American Academy of Osteopathy, Colorado, Colorado Springs, 1937).

12. Stoner, F. *The Eclectic Approach to Chiropractice* (FLS Publishing Co., Las Vegas, 1977).

13. *Which*, Consumer Association Report on Alternative Medicine (October 1986).

14. Inglis, B. and West, R. *The Alternative Health Guide* (Michael Joseph, London, 1983), pp. 116–18.

15. Pearson, D. and Shaw, S. *Life Extension* (Warner Books, New York, 1982), p. 6.

USEFUL ADDRESSES

'Touch for Health'
39 Browns Road
Surbiton
Surrey
KT5 8ST
Telephone: 01 399 3215

(Associated Societies: Touch for Health Foundation in California, USA, also British Touch for Health Association)

7

The Alexander Technique:
Postural Re-education for Health

Sue Thame

INTRODUCTION

When I was invited to contribute a chapter to this book I hesitated because I wondered whether the Alexander technique could rightly be termed a complementary therapy. There seems to be a popular, if mistaken, perception that the technique is part of 'alternative' medicine, and I feared the inclusion of an article on the technique in this book would further promote that mistaken view. Alexander always took care to place his work within *education* not *medicine*. Practitioners of the technique have always followed his lead, calling themselves teachers rather than therapists. People come to them for lessons, not for treatment.

Complementary medicine takes a holistic view, seeing the patient's resources as integral to the healing process, with the therapist as the expert assistant, bringing specialist knowledge and experience to help the patient heal himself. This view of the central role of the patient marries closely with the educational perspective that the technique follows. It suggests that people improve their functioning, at whatever level — mental, emotional and physical — through their own efforts and wishes, and with the assistance of skilful teachers. The Alexander technique specifically sets out to improve the functioning of a person's mind and body in movement. This is known as 'psychophysical re-education'.

For nurses, whose work is intensely physical, the technique offers special help in their day-to-day work of bending, lifting and carrying. It shows how they can protect themselves from injury and strain while providing effective services to patients. If they are aware of the principles of the technique they can also improve the way they assist patients to cope with the distress and tensions of being bed-bound or incapacitated in whatever way. In many circumstances of recovery from illnesses — for example, back pain and related disorders, breathing and vocal disorders, muscular dysfunctions, and with some disabilities like spasticity — the technique has a history of helpful cooperation with medical treatment. This chapter aims to show the complementary nature of the teaching of the Alexander technique with healing.

THE BASIC PRINCIPLES OF THE ALEXANDER TECHNIQUE

Definitions

From a medical perspective, the technique can be seen as preventive postural health care. As this is a simple definition there is an immediate danger that its simplicity will mislead the reader to think that the technique is just posture-training, because it is not generally recognised that posture is a highly significant contributor to health. The focus of the technique makes posture central in health care. This idea can be illustrated by drawing on a concept used in the technique, referred to as the unity of psychophysical functioning.

In the Alexander technique it is suggested that the habitual stance of the body is said to reveal habitual attitudes of the mind. Health and sickness arise from the complex interweaving of the mind and body in which long-term habitual patterns of behaviour play the major part. If people wish to change their unhealthy psychological states they will also have to change their physical states. Conversely, if they wish to change their unhealthy postures, they will also have to change some of their patterns of thinking. Posture is regarded as the manifestation of mind and thus intimately linked with health.

Making changes in posture is not easy. Simple instructions to 'stand upright', 'bend properly', 'walk tall', 'go jogging', and 'swim regularly' are not adequate. These supposedly remedial activities will all be carried out within the overall deep habit patterns of movement unconsciously absorbed in childhood which are usually counter to good poise. Because these habits are unconscious, special training for poised, balanced and integrated movement is therefore required. To understand the intricacies, difficulties and subtleties of this kind of posture-training it is necessary to be aware of what is involved when a person embarks on changing the habits of a lifetime.

Habits of movement are usually so unseen and unknown to the individual that should they catch a glimpse of themselves walking by a shop window they may not recognise themselves. It is often distressing to people when they see themselves for the first time moving on video. Usually they have no idea how they move and they are shocked to discover that their internal image of what they look like when they move is quite different from reality. What is even more distressing though is that if they want to change or correct their characteristic movement patterns, they do not have a conscious process they can use that will bring a satisfactory result.

The movements of the body have their origins in the silent and unseen movements of mind, both conscious and unconscious, of which people are largely unaware. What the technique can do is provide the process to integrate mind and body in dynamic movement, raise these dynamics to consciousness and show what kind of learning is needed in order to replace old, ill-adapted movement patterns with new. The emphasis of the technique is on 'human learning' in the process of physical activity.

DEVELOPMENT OF THE TECHNIQUE

Background

The originator of the technique, Frederick Matthias Alexander was born in Tasmania in 1869 and spent most of his adult teaching life in England and the United States. Alexander's biography reveals him to be an outstanding man with an individualistic approach. The development of his technique arose from a personal quest to resolve his own vocal problems which were preventing him from fulfilling his ambition to become a successful Shakespearean actor. He undertook years of patient, lonely and highly original research, without any formal scientific tutoring, to arrive at the central concepts of his technique which, in a phrase, deal with the proper psychophysical coordination of the human being.

Long after his death his research was significantly recognised by Nikolaas Tinbergen, when he gave his Nobel prizewinning speech in Stockholm, Sweden, in December 1973. In his speech Tinbergen drew the links between his own scientific approach as an ethnologist and Alexander's observational methods.[1]

In the 1880s and 1890s, when Alexander carried out his

fundamental research, he was working within the explosion of interest in the theory of evolution. It enabled him to set his individual discoveries within the context of an evolutionary understanding of man's development. He established that he was exploring the development of man's conscious thinking over instinctive responses and the disruptive effects this appeared to have on our psychological and physical functioning in a modern civilisation. He widened his field into health and education and in 1904 the Australian medical profession encouraged him to go to England to make his work known to a wider public.

He built a successful practice which attracted people who wanted to both learn and teach the technique. Gradually he developed a unique style in which the use of touch played an important role. Communicating this skill with the hands to others required many years of patient experiment and development. From the 1920s to his death in 1955 he continued to explore and refine his teaching methods. Today the use of touch has become an important aspect of the Alexander technique. Since his death Alexander teachers liaise and cooperate with many complementary therapies.

The qualification of teachers is supervised by a professional body, the Society of Teachers of the Alexander Technique (STAT), based in London, who award certificates of teaching after a three-year full-time training. This Society ensures that only properly trained and qualified practitioners can call themselves teachers of the Alexander Technique.

The technique and health care

Many patients' ailments arise from, or are aggravated by, the postural misuse of their bodies.

Replacement surgery can in some cases substitute new parts for old. But this is expensive and not always satisfactory. However, it is a long-accepted canon in health care that it is more effective to prevent than to cure or treat. This is a view with which the Alexander technique fully agrees and tries to put into practice as a primary concern. It seeks to teach people how to become proficient in the care of their own body mechanics.

But if this were all, the technique would not be particularly distinctive. There are physiotherapists, doctors, osteopaths, athletics coaches, teachers of the performing arts, yoga teachers and many other skilled specialists who teach body-care mechanics. What distinguishes the Alexander teacher is twofold: first, the way of approaching the human side of body-mechanics management — that is, the conscious and unconscious learning processes involved; and second, a system-wide understanding of how the human body optimally functions in movement. These two distinctive aspects of the technique are detailed a little later when discussing what is taught in the technique.

The technique as re-education

A principal concern for the Alexander teacher is the learning that individuals have to undertake if they are to improve their skills of body movement. Learning has to take place in the context of the individual's lifestyle, job, responsibilities and ambitions. What is distinctive about this learning is that it is a 're-education', involving mind and heart as well as the body. Perhaps this word 're-education' needs to be spelled out for its significance to come through. 'Education' is taken to mean the process whereby young people and adults learn something for the first time — skills of one kind and another that are new to them. 'Re-education' is a process of correction needed when people have learned skills inaccurately, when they do not do them well, and when they need to attain higher standards of skilfulness.

Re-education is difficult. A learned, incorrect skill is much harder to change and improve to a new standard than starting afresh to reach the same standard. It is far better to ensure that a child or adult learns something *right* in the first place. Learning it wrong in the first place then requires having to unlearn what is wrong before learning what is right. Nurses and health care workers frequently face similar problems when attempting to change a part of a patient's habitual lifestyle, like smoking, which is detrimental to their health.

It is the re-education process that is at the heart of the technique and this is the process that Alexander teachers offer help with. Their skills are related specifically to changing the fundamental, generic patterns of learned body movements which adversely affect every single human activity — sitting, talking, walking, bending, writing, reading, laughing, crying, lifting, running, listening, watching TV — the list is endless. Most people in the western world today make their daily movements unskilfully, in ways they picked up subconsciously as children. While many of the movements in themselves may not seem to be dramatically damaging to the wear

103

and tear of the body, over the prolonged period of a lifetime, each badly executed movement takes its toll physically and psychologically. The backbone usually suffers most. Knee joints, and shoulder joints are close runners-up.

What is not generally recognised, but significantly addressed by the technique, is the toll that poor posture takes on the mind. The inner self suffers from prolonged postural imbalance. In addition we are also influenced by visual and social influences such as ungraceful attitudes, postures and movements that are adopted by people during daily activities. In this respect, the visual impact which nurses make upon their patients as they go about their daily work in the wards may be a valuable teaching aid.

WHAT IS TAUGHT IN THE TECHNIQUE

Teaching the Alexander technique involves a two-sided approach — understanding the dynamics of movement, and human learning. In the context of the written word here we are limited to a linear approach which means we have to read one idea after another rather than view both simultaneously. This is a problem which always seems to hamper explanations of anything that purports to be holistic and which, by definition, cannot be wholly described by reductionist analysis, that is by splitting it up to examine it. Other media such as arts, images, drama, and poetry seem far more appropriate for conveying the holistic messages than does written prose.

In the past Alexander teachers have had a certain notoriety in their refusals to write about the technique due to their belief that readers would be gulled into thinking that they had experienced and understood the technique merely by reading about it. For similar reasons Alexander himself only wrote four major books (listed at the end of the chapter). He constantly warned against the danger of assuming that because you have read about something you therefore understand it. Consequently one of the hallmarks of the technique is practical practice. Teachers learn their trade by doing it under intensive tuition. I estimate that 80 per cent of the Alexander teacher's three years of training is practical work.

The practical knowledge of body dynamics

The core idea of the technique's approach to body dynamics was first unravelled by Alexander in the 1880s and 1890s through a series of remarkable studies painstakingly described in his book *The Use of the Self*.[2] This offers a detailed picture of Alexander's central concept of body dynamics which he called the 'primary control'. Alexander discovered, by careful empirical research, that the balance or poise of the head on top of the torso governs the quality of the whole movement-pattern of the body.[2] He discerned that undue tension in the head–neck–back musculature had implications for the good coordination of the rest of the body. The movement of the body, plus the quality of 'released', un-tense moving, is controlled through headbalance. He perceived that movement begins from the head. The fundamental integrity of movement in the human body is thus dependent upon the head–neck–torso relationship. Subsequent research has verified Alexander's findings.[3]

Integrity and interference

What then is the nature of this head–neck–torso integrity and how is it interefered with? First let us deal with integrity of movement. It is important to recognise that we are not dealing with static posture, but with dynamic balance. The head weighs anywhere between 4.5–6.3 kg (10–14 lbs) and is in constant motion. It appears as an unstable ball resting insecurely on the articular facets of the atlas. The leverage effected by the head on top of the long body of the upright human means that our balance is highly unstable. It would seem, however, that we have developed a marked tendency in our culture to reduce that dynamic instability through tensing our musculature around the head and neck and shortening our whole stature. This tendency seems to have become endemic.

Contrast for example western posture with the elegance of the native Indian, who can carry 13½ kg (30 lbs) on the head without stress. Alexander put our loss of physical integrity down to city life, to prolonged 'indoors' living, to too much sitting in chairs, haste, and to the development of intellect and reasoning which overruled instincts without substituting adequate conscious control. The natural integrity of the human body, indeed for all vertebrates, is dependent upon a freely poised head, a minimum necessary tension in the head–neck–torso and a lengthened musculature and expanded structure from head to toe when moving.

Alexander argued that interference of this natural integrity diminished the functioning of the proprioceptors. Our sense of movement comes through the kinaesthetic movement receptors. The richness of the sense of movement is, therefore, dependent upon the

Figure 7.1: The optimal position of head and neck for adequate balance

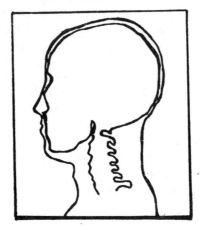

full and free movement of joints where receptors are clustered. Joints that are tightened through tension inhibit receptors from firing, thus reducing the information about movement to the brain. Where this is most significant is in the neck which has the richest concentrations of receptors. Stiffness in the neck can diminish the information flow about movement to the brain.

It is also an area where people most frequently complain of stiffness and tension. The principal cause is a difficulty in balancing the heavy weight of the head which has its centre of gravity forward and up from the point of balance at the atlanto-occipital joint (Figure 7.1).

While this form of headbalance has its purposes (the main one being to ensure that the forward-inclining head is always gently stretching the neck, exciting the receptors to fire, thus stimulating constant information about the movement of the head on the neck to enliven balance) in our western civilisation our kinaesthetic sense of headbalance has become debased. We lock our heads onto our necks, for whatever reasons, stiffening our neck joints (Figure 7.2).

By doing this we impair not only the balance of the head but also the balance of the whole body. Tensing the head on the body is a subtle activity. If it is to be corrected and incorporated into the complexities of an individual's daily life it requires refined methods of correction. The Alexander technique has developed just such methods, described in the next section.

Figure 7.2: A commonly adopted position of the head and neck whereby the head is 'locked' onto the neck. This causes an imbalance of the head and neck which can also affect the balance of the whole body

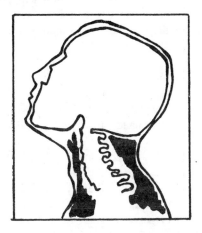

Learning how to change unwanted habits

There are three stages in the learning process.

(1) Raising to consciousness the habitual movement patterns of the head–neck–torso (primary control) in all their manifestations.
(2) 'Inhibiting' or preventing the spontaneous repetition of those habits.
(3) Deciding what new pattern of primary control is desired and how to carry it out.

Let us take these three stages of learning in the context of an Alexander lesson, to reveal how the teacher sets about the task.

The typical lesson would be conducted in a teaching room in which there is a chair, full-length mirror and a firm working-table. Lessons for a more advanced pupil might well be given outdoors or in a special situation — for example, during tennis, piano playing, acting, golf, etc. Some early steps in learning only are given here. Initially the pupil or patient, has to become aware of the central significance of head poise. Telling the pupil will, of course, create an immediate intellectual understanding. But we are looking for a practical understanding of what it means. So the teacher might invite the

107

pupil to sit down in the chair and stand up again. Asked 'What did you do with your head?' the pupil might look puzzled and reply that he/she hadn't a clue. That is the nub of the problem. The untutored person has little conscious experience of the balance of head as he/she moves. Without that consciousness he/she cannot judge effectively whether the balance is well-managed or not.

The three stages of learning

At this juncture the Alexander teacher can highlight the head balance through the use of his/her hands. Inviting the pupil to sit down again, the teacher might place his/her hands on the pupil's head, particularly at the head–neck axis. Immediately the pupil's consciousness of his/her own head is raised. The sensory experience of touching hands reveals to him/her what they are doing to his/her head. He/she often finds that it is jerked back and down each time he/she sits down and gets up again. Repetition of this procedure further reveals to the pupil that he/she does not know how to change this habit. The misuse of the head in this way hugely disturbs the whole body balance, causing the back to shorten and stiffen, and the arms to tighten, and initiates tension in the thighs, calves and feet.

During the second stage the teacher shows the pupil how to 'inhibit' or prevent these wrong movements. Usually this can be assisted by a combination of skilful support through the hands and focused mental work until the pupil can 'sense' the moment the impulse to do the wrong action actually takes place. This is the moment to 'inhibit', to pause so that the intention to move is held back. At this point the teacher introduces the third stage — new directions for control of the balance of the head in relation to the whole body. Not only must the head movement change but all the associated tension patterns throughout the body must also be released. This is referred to as 'giving directions'.

The movements that are being examined must be slowed down in order to learn how to release muscle tension. Every thought carries a reciprocal muscle tension, and these linkages must be unwound. One of the favoured ways in the technique is through 'lying-down work' on the working-table. The pupil takes up a semisupine position, with head supported by a small pile of books in order to maintain the integrity of the head–neck–torso relationship. Then the teacher moves the pupil's head, arms and legs, encouraging the release of muscle tension and giving the experience of movement in the limbs without tension. This releases the joints, promotes a richer experience of the proprioceptors, and enlivens the pupil's sense of movement. He/she begins to experience movement as a 'sensation' rather than simply an 'action'. It may even change his/her experience of time and may cause him/her to confront his/her deeply unconscious 'hurry-up' intentions, which impel him/her to execute all movements in haste, ensuring continuous, never-released muscle tension. Alexander called this haste 'end-gaining', seeing it as western man's most prevalent psychological illness.

Applying the principles in all of life

When the basic principles of the technique have been learned in standing up and sitting down, the pupil will be ready to extend his/her range, to learn how to make the primary control function effective in all his/her activities. Here the teacher can provide support through physical touch similar to the earlier psychophysical training. The pupil gradually learns to apply the principles involved in the movements of sitting and standing to *all* bending activities. The learning process can then progress to twisting, walking and all locomotor activities, manual dexterity and to reading and visual activity.

People usually experience their lessons as freeing and releasing occasions, bringing them more in touch with themselves as they grow more in touch with their bodies. People report, for example, that they have more energy, move more freely, feel better in their bodies, manage stress better, and have more stamina in work. The physical touching from the teacher can in itself be healing. There will be times, of course, when nothing seems to be changing, and the pupil feels stuck. A break, a period of reflection may be necessary, or the assistance of other therapists may be required. I have gladly involved the help of osteopaths, acupuncturists, reflexologists, herbalists and counsellors with my pupils. Finding the way through habits is a complex business, requiring many different skills.

THE LINKS WITH COMPLEMENTARY AND ORTHODOX MEDICINE

Sir George Trevelyan, a leading advocate and pioneer of alternative approaches in education and health, was awakened to the Alexander technique in the 1930s, when he trained as a teacher with Alexander himself. In the early 1980s, on one of his visits to the London-based Alexander technique training centre (the Alexander Teaching Associates), he spoke of the technique as a foundation skill for everyone in health care.[4] All health care workers meet with inordinate physical and mental stresses when helping people. Their bodies are the instruments through which they carry out their work. The manner of their 'use', whether good or poor, and the patterns of thinking that are manifested in their postures, will be part of the interplay in their physical and emotional relationship with their patients.

How does the technique help nurses and health care workers?

One of the most important effects of the practice of the Alexander technique is the means it provides for health care workers to bring themselves into balance within themselves and towards other people. It enables them to improve the quality of health care that they give. Let us take a straightforward example; other people's suffering and pain can drain energy from the nurse, who is constantly bending to do physical work, listen and talk to patients. How he/she bends will affect how much energy is expended emotionally and physically. Using the technique staff can manage ways of responding with greater awareness of the effects of bending on themselves and on their patients. He/she will be able to sustain his/her effective care to high standards without tiring so much. A further effect will be on their quality of touch. Having a better sense of how to maintain the integrity of one's body will generate less tension in the arms and hands. For the sick person touch becomes a healing agent of great importance.

What if the nurse, midwife, or doctor are themselves in pain? For many conditions the technique is an available adjunct to medical care. A London doctor told me that he had found that the technique enabled him to keep his sciatic pain at bay. Although treatments of physiotherapy, acupuncture, tablets, swimming and rest also helped, the technique gave him a means, while he was actually working, to ensure that he moved in ways that would not activate his problem. A dentist who had severe back pain that could not be resolved by orthodox or complementary medical methods, in desperation and deep scepticism turned to the technique. It enabled him to 'manage' the pain. He said it took time to overcome his scepticism that re-education of his body would make a difference; but with regular lessons he has been able to get back to work.

When people are in pain, as these two examples show, the technique's concept that 'use affects functioning' comes vividly alive. When you have pain arising from, for example the back, movements that are poorly executed will be far more painful than movements carried out with good primary control, that is good 'use' of the self. People in pain tend to tense themselves even more than usual; they really should release their tension to assist the healing process. The technique helps them to reverse their 'natural' tensing reaction to pain. There are, of course, many Alexander pupils, both medical and lay, who can testify to this. In 1985, a London hospital piloted a programme to experiment with a number of therapies for pain management. One Alexander teacher, who has congenital hip malformation and a long biography of pain and surgical operations from childhood, was invited to contribute. After completion, her contribution on the Alexander technique was given top rating by patients' preferences at the three-month follow-up.[5] The programme is running again this year, with continued Alexander work.

Preventive health care

One group of medical practitioners who have been consistently interested in the application of the technique in their work are physiotherapists. A number of Alexander teachers working in the United Kingdom today are also physiotherapists and they have encouraged 'cross-fertilisation'. A current programme underway, led by an Alexander teacher who is also a chartered physiotherapist, provides evening classes for physiotherapists. One major aim is to help physiotherapists take better care of their *own* bodies while they give treatment, and learn to improve their own kinaesthetic appreciation of how they move. This heightens their awareness of their own habit patterns which interfere with good functioning. Their second aim is to examine how patients, who repeatedly strain themselves, can be re-educated so that they can prevent future recurrences. The physiotherapists will become better teachers because of their better self-awareness.[6]

Physiotherapists try to provide preventive health care for people who have already made themselves ill. With children, in particular, it is better to do it before they get ill. Surrey County Council, with the encouragement of the Back Pain Association, has supported Alexander work through experimental programmes in first and middle schools and with inservice training for teachers. They have also produced a video[7] showing how the technique might be used to help children better appreciate the 'use' of their growing bodies. I worked closely with Surrey County Council throughout this project (1978–82), and saw for myself how the conditions in schools interfere with children's development of good postural use of their bodies.

A valuable PhD research project is now nearing completion, called 'Posture education with the primary school physical education curriculum with special reference to the Alexander technique'. This has been carried out by a physical educationalist, John Handley,[8] who has been investigating the benefits of the Alexander technique in schooling. It is hoped that a teacher's manual is to be developed from this, to be used in inservice training for a new programme of posture training in primary schools. The Health Education Council (HEC) have also incorporated elements of Alexander's posture model into their project 'Look after Yourself'.

The Back Pain Association has invited Mr Handley to join a working party which is focusing on education. Mr Handley comments that it would not be difficult to introduce certain Alexander principles into teacher training programmes and into training of school nurses and, it is hoped, schools of general nursing. He says:

> Teachers need to understand that body-use is affected by the mind as well as by the design and dimensions of the furniture. Using one's body with the minimum amount of muscular effort is a psychomotor skill. The earlier this skill development programme is implemented the easier it is to extinguish incorrect learned habits.[8]

Teacher-training today

There are approximately 1000 trained teachers of the Alexander technique around the world. Not all teachers register with the Society of Teachers of the Alexander Technique (STAT), but it is useful to be able to check qualifications through the Society. Numbers of teachers are growing rapidly as new training schools are established and as the demand for Alexander work increases. The experience of most teachers is that public interest and desire for lessons is spreading, supported by the media and word-of-mouth recommendation.

In the period of rapid growth of the 1970s and 1980s, there has been concern within STAT about maintenance of teaching standards. We are well aware of the need to raise standards, to widen the curriculum to incorporate the latest medical and educational findings, while preserving what is essential from the past. Students are dogged by financial burdens because there are only very limited local authority grants in the United Kingdom. Foreign students are able to obtain educational loans and grants far more readily. This, of course, affects the provision of training facilities, the types of people who come forward as students, and the remuneration of teachers who give the training. The effect is largely positive. People who enter for training are highly motivated, having overcome many obstacles. Teachers who work in training schools are dedicated, with many years' experience.

Having lessons today

In order to learn the technique for your own benefit one has to be prepared to give it some time. Different teachers recommend different time-arrangements. Some suggest up to three half-hour lessons a week initially, to establish the basics. Others prefer a longer lesson of an hour at a time, once a week, so the pupil can gain some extended experience of putting the technique into practice between lessons. How many lessons a pupil takes to get a good grounding varies and will depend on his circumstances. Some people are immediately responsive, perhaps because they have studied and experienced other good generic disciplines like tai-chi or yoga, and they are often able to make connections quickly and grasp the principles with ease. Others find it quite alien and even resent the expectation that they must work with the technique for themselves if they are to benefit from it. In these cases it is the skill of the teacher that helps them take responsibility.

CONCLUSIONS

If the Alexander technique work is to be successful it can only be with the active responsibility of the pupil for his own learning and development. In speaking to many colleagues and pupils in preparation for writing this chapter, I found they were consistent in their emphasis on this. A colleague who is a practising Alexander teacher and dentist told me that he endeavours to bring the same principles of self-responsibility into his dentistry, by teaching preventive dental health care.[9]

The Alexander technique offers tremendous potential to all nurses and health care workers in their own self-care not only in preventing back disorders caused by incorrect posture and lifting of patients, but also in the relief of stress, tension and a heightened awareness of health as the mutual interdependence of the mind and the body. The Director of the school where I was trained once remarked: 'If you are getting nowhere look first into yourself; look for the cause within yourself and your own possible mis-use. Only then, if you can find no impediment, do you look to the cause in your pupil'.[10]

Holistic health begins within each one of us — we must try to keep our own house in order while caring for others.

NOTES AND REFERENCES

1. Tinbergen, 'Ethology and Stress Disease', *Science* (1974), 185, pp. 20–27.

2. Alexander, F.M. *The Use of the Self* (London, Integral Press, 1932).

3. Coghill, G.E. 'Appreciation: The Educational Methods of F. Matthias Alexander', in Alexander, F.M. *The Universal Constant in Living* (Dutton, New York, 1941, 3rd printing 1942).

4. Sir George Trevelyan Bt, MA, former principal of Attingham Park, a pioneering centre for adult education (1948–71). In his retirement he now undertakes speaking commitments on all aspects of healing of body, mind and spirit in Britain and abroad. He can be contacted at The Old Vicarage, Hawkesbury, near Badminton, Gloucestershire GL9 1BN.

5. Unpublished report of Royal National Orthopaedic Hospital's Pain Management Programme. The section on the Alexander Technique was written by Liz Scanell, who can be contacted through the Society of Teachers of the Alexander Technique.

6. Carmen Burton, Member of the Chartered Society of the Physiotherapy and Teaching Member of STAT has led programmes at the Royal Orthopaedic Hospital, the Oxford Group of Hospitals, the National Hospital for Nervous Diseases, and Charing Cross Hospital. Mrs Burton can be contacted via the Society of Teachers of the Alexander Technique.

7. Thame, S. *Saving Yourself from Stress* (Media Resources Centre, Ewell, Surrey, 1981). Videotapes also available from Surrey Media Resources Centre, Glyn House, Church Street, Ewell, Surrey, UK.

8. Handley, J. *Posture Education within the Primary School Physical Education Curriculum with Special Reference to the Alexander Technique*

(unpublished thesis, London University Institute of Education, London, 1986).

9. Barry Collins, BDS, dental surgeon and Alexander teacher. He can be contacted via the Society of Teachers of the Alexander Technique.

10. Walter Carrington, Director of Constructive Teaching Centre; author's reported recollection of his lecture to students.

BOOKS, ARTICLES AND SOURCES OF INFORMATION

Books

Alexander, F.M. *Man's Supreme Inheritance* (Manchester, Re-educational Publications Ltd, 1910).

Alexander, F.M. *Constructive Conscious Control of the Individual* (London, Methuen and Co. Ltd, 1923).

Alexander, F.M. *The Use of the Self* (Integral Press, London, 1932).

Alexander, F.M. *The Universal Constant in Living* (Dutton, New York, 1941).

Barlow, W. *The Alexander Principle* (Victor Gollancz, London, also in paperback, Arrow). A doctor's description of the technique.

Carrington, W.H.M. 'The F. Matthias Alexander Technique: A Means of Understanding Man', *Systematics*, vol. 1 (4) (March, 1963).

Carrington, W.H.M. *Man's Future as an Individual* (Sheldrake Press, London, 1969).

Dart, R. *An Anatomist's Tribute to F. Matthias Alexander* (Sheldrake Press, London, 1970).

Fenton, J.V. *Choice of Habit* (Macdonald Evans Ltd, London, 1973). Tells how a headmaster introduced the Alexander technique into schools.

Gelb, M. *Body Learning: An Introduction to the Alexander Technique* (Aurum Press, London, 1981).

Jones, F.P. *Body Awareness in Action. A Study of the Alexander Technique* (Schocken Books, New York, 1976).

Jones, F.P. *Learning How to Learn: An Operational Definition of the Alexander Technique* (Sheldrake Press, London, 1974).

Thame, S. *The Alexander Technique for Stress* (Joint Development Resources, Pinner, Middlesex, 1984).

Articles

Dart, R.A. 'The Postural Aspect of Malocclusion', in the official *Journal of the DASA South Africa*, (1946) 1 (1).

Dart, R.A. 'The Attainment of Poise'. *South African Medical Journal* (8 February 1947).

Magnus, R. (1925) *Animal Posture* Croonian Lecture. *Proceedings of the Royal Society Series B*, 98 (1925).

Some recommended pamphlets are available from the Constructive Teaching Centre, 18 Lansdown Road, London W11 3LL.

Courses

Information on public courses (some residential) are available from:

Alexander Teaching Centre, 188 Old St, London EC1V 9BP
Constructive Teaching Centre, 18 Lansdowne Rd, London W11 3LL
Gill and Mike Birley, 37 Park Lane, Norwich, Norfolk NR2 3EF
Jenny Daisley, 103 Salisbury Rd, London W13 9TT
Bob Donovan, 14 Saxon Rd, Winchester, Hants SE23 7DS
Alan Mars and Refia Sacks, 137 Grosvenor Avenue, Highbury, London N5
Jamie McDowell and Francien Schoonens, 9 St Mark's Rise, London E8 2NJ

The list is not exhaustive. There are many courses being run with specialist needs in mind (for example, for young musicians); contact Mrs Elizabeth Waterhouse, 86 Cromwell Avenue, Highgate, London N6 5HQ. Details of courses may be found by telephoning the Alexander teacher in your area or by contacting STAT, or any one of the teaching schools.

USEFUL ADDRESS

The Society of Teachers of the Alexander Technique (STAT)
10 London House
266 Fulham Road
London SW10 9EL

Details of teachers in the United Kingdom and abroad and of training schools will be sent on request.

8

Massage

Allan Mason

INTRODUCTION

For the last 150 years or so, western medicine has tended to be dominated by a mechanistic concept of biology.[1] Individuals have frequently come to be seen as a conglomeration of parts and processes, and 'illness' as any deviation from some predetermined pattern of chemical formulae or numerical values. In this reductionist perspective, the patient tends to be thought of as a machine. This approach contrasts with the holistic health care perspective which maintains that the patient represents more than the sum of these parts alone.

It would appear that there is a present trend for both practitioners and patients to turn away from the reductionist model of illness towards a more holistic approach to health care which acknowledges the potential influence of social, psychological and spiritual factors in experience of disease and disability.[2]

One of the oldest and simplest forms of physical remedy employing an holistic approach to health and illness is massage. In the formal sense it is usually associated with the deliberate and purposeful manipulations that are a part of professional practice, while informally it can be taken to include the vigorous rubbing of an injured part, or the gentle stroking that eases pain and anxiety.

Observation, clinical experience and research have all indicated that massage can produce a variety of physical and physiological effects — for example, an increase in circulation, reduction of swelling, altered muscle flexibility and changes in autonomic activity.[3] This has made it an effective treatment of choice in sports medicine[4] and in the management of severely scarred soft tissues.[5] It is, perhaps, a truism to state that a sense of touch is necessary for the practice of massage; but many do not realise that it is through this important sense that the holistic implications of care can be appreciated and understood.

In the human animal, touch plays a vital role in the development and maintenance of the 'haptic system'. This is a term that was coined by Gibson[6] to denote the 'sensibility of the individual to the world adjacent to his body, by the use of his body'. It represents a person's model of the world constructed in order to make sense of and to act within it. This model is organised around the sense of touch and the giving and receiving of physical contact.

A baby tries to make sense of the outside world by directly experiencing its physical reality. Later, he learns to translate that experience into concepts and abstractions of adult existence.[7] For example, words such as 'sharp' or 'wet' subsume a wealth of investigative knowledge and, generally speaking, require no primary confirmation of their meaning. First-hand experience, however, becomes important whenever reality cannot be wholly defined through language — for example, squeezing an ofange to test its ripeness, or feeling the quality of a piece of material.

While touching the world is important in the establishment or confirmation of reality, the experience of being touched is vital to the way that the individual sees or interprets that reality. A baby's early introduction to the experience of being held and cuddled gives him a measure of security in a strange and frightening world. The extent and quality of touching that he receives will largely determine his view of the world and of his part in it.[8-10] Through the giving and receiving of contact, a child begins to build up a picture of what is in the world and what it means to him as an individual. He gradually integrates these elements into a flexible and harmonious system that allows for adjustment to the changes in fortune, circumstance and environment that are part of life. Once the child has entered the 'adult world of concepts' he can relegate touch to a minor role. Language tends to replace primary tactile experience, and 'cuddling' is directed into socially acceptable codes of behaviour. However, when there is a serious threat to the integrity of the individual — for example, after amputation of a limb, spinal paralysis, or during periods of extreme stress, the haptic system may not be able to make the necessary adjustment if personal resources are overstressed. The system must be slowly and painfully rebuilt to take into consideration a different reality. It can be said that the sense of touch can significantly aid the process of haptic restructuring.

Massage, because of its physical effects on the body, and its role in haptic restructuring, can provide a 'whole person' approach to the many problems of disease, dysfunction and disability.

THE HISTORY AND DEVELOPMENT OF MASSAGE

Massage in one form or another has been used by a wide variety of medical systems in a broad spectrum of cultures and civilisations. There is evidence to suppose that it was known in China, India and by the physicians of ancient Greece and Rome.[11] Its history as a legitimate therapeutic remedy has, however, been frequently accompanied by the notion that it is the trademark of the quack or the charlatan. Consequently massage can be seen in all levels of practice ranging from medical orthodoxy to traditional folk medicine and the massage parlour.

It may be more useful to think of the development of modern massage through the influence of 19th century practitioners. The formal presentation of massage can be attributed to the work of Metzger in Holland,[11] and Ling in Sweden.[12] Their work was, in part, a contribution to the revival of interest in 'natural therapies' which were centred around massage, gymnastics and electrotherapy, and also extended to include diet and the use of air, water and sunlight for the promotion of health.

By the 1880s there were a number of people, mostly women, who were giving massage treatments under the authority of physicians for a variety of medical complaints. By this time the Weir Mitchell regime was popular in Great Britain. This was devised by a Philadelphia physician and consisted of long periods of rest and isolation interspersed with sessions of massage and electricity. It was prescribed for those patients who were exhausted by the 'rush of modern life' and who were labelled neurasthenic (pp. 579–83).[12]

In 1895 a small group of nurses who were employed as 'medical rubbers' in London hospitals decided to form a society of massage to establish standards of practice. The Society of Trained Masseuses as it was called subsequently became the Chartered Society of Massage and Medical Gymnastics in 1920, and in 1942 it adopted its present title of the Chartered Society of Physiotherapy.

The original society was built around the practice of Swedish massage, and this continues to be taught to present-day physiotherapy students. There has, however, been one fairly recent development in massage technique known as 'connective tissue massage'. This has evolved from the empirical work of Elizabeth Dicke,[13] and her massage techniques have been developed by Ebner[14] as a formal therapeutic method.

The use of massage outside the physiotherapeutic field is, however, considerable and can be seen in three broad categories of work:

(1) In remedial therapy by practitioners who are not eligible for state registration and whose training schools may not be liable to independent inspection or supervision. This may include practitioners with little or no training at all.
(2) In beauty therapy where massage is taught as part of a wider course that is cosmetic rather than strictly medical.
(3) In psychotherapy where some therapists advocate the use of massage as one strategy in behaviour analysis and treatment.[9] Massage is often used in the field of 'growth and awareness', and when carried out by responsible professionals in a controlled environment can play a vital role in health care practice.

THE TECHNIQUES OF MASSAGE

Basic massage manoeuvres are fairly easy to learn as they represent natural movements of the hands. Most individuals can give a pleasant and acceptable massage, but while the manipulations themselves can be understood from descriptions or pictures, there are many aspects of massage that cannot be learnt from books — for example, how hard to press, what normal tissues feel like, or whether technical variations are appropriate. It takes some training and a great deal of practice to achieve an efficient and therapeutically effective level of practice. There are, however, a number of guidelines that underlie massage and it is important that these are understood, since massage is as much an approach as it is a series of manoeuvres or techniques. These guidelines can be described under three broad headings: environment, patient/model, and operator/therapist.

GUIDELINES FOR SUCCESSFUL MASSAGE

Environment

The room that is being used should be warm and comfortable, bearing in mind that the person being massaged will have to remove some of his clothing. Harsh lighting should be avoided wherever possible and overhead lights may be particularly uncomfortable to the eyes when a person is lying on his back. Couches or beds must be firm without being unduly hard, and covered with a blanket or sheet. Any apparatus should be placed within easy reach so that the flow of massage is not disrupted.

Patient/model

He or she should be in a comfortable position, well supported with pillows. It is best to choose a position that can be maintained for the duration of the massage. Clothing must be removed from the area being massaged and the rest of the body covered with a sheet if necessary.

Operator/therapist

He or she must be physically and mentally relaxed. It is too easy to communicate a state of mind or body to another person by the physical contact that is made. The operator must create a 'healing' effect in which the patient/model feels secure and at ease. This means that the operator must, to some extent, merge with the background and not allow his/her person, dress or voice to become prominent or obtrusive.

Hands

These form the most important element in massage. They should be clean, with short nails, not too cold or hot and sweaty. It is a good idea to wash the hands in cool water and then to do a few stretching exercises to enliven the circulation. No rings should be worn as these may well catch on the skin. It is helpful for the operator to spend just a few moments 'centring', that is, becoming mentally relaxed and concentrating on the task in hand.

MASSAGE MEDIUM

Either powder or oil can be used. Talcum powder makes a very effective medium for massage but it must be mild and unscented. Very little is needed and it should be lightly dusted over the hands, never over the patient. Under certain conditions, oil can be used in massage and this is particularly useful when the skin is dry or flaky, for example when a limb has just come out of plaster. Oil, however, tends to be a messy medium and its slippery nature limits the number of techniques that can be used; if it is used, however, a bland baby oil is preferable.

THE MASSAGE

Posture

Both model and operator must be comfortable. From the operator's point of view a poor posture makes massage very tiring and will give rise to aching muscles and fatigue. Weight should be evenly distributed over both feet.

Hand movements

These must be firm and purposeful. Massage should never be half-hearted or the movements 'fidgety'. The hands should move like water over the skin, moulding to every contour of the body, but remaining in total contact.

There should always be a smooth change from one manoeuvre to another so that there is never an awareness of change only a sense of continuity. There are three basic manipulations to consider in massage — stroking, kneading and striking.

Basic manipulations

Stroking

The hands are placed on the part to be massaged and then moved slowly and rhythmically in the direction of the venous drainage of the limb or body. If venous return is not a prime consideration, then stroking can be done in any direction. Pressure can be light or deep and the rate quick or slow — but it must, at all times, be consistent and rhythmical.

This is a good technique for increasing the venous and lymphatic drainage from the periphery, and for stimulating circulation. At the same time, it helps the operator to become familiar with the details of the tissues, their texture, contours, levels of tension or relaxation, and with the presence of lumps, bumps or nodules. Stroking is also used as a transitional stroke linking different manipulations.

Kneading

This technique will move the skin on muscle, muscle on muscle or tissue on tissue. It must, therefore, be firm and definitive. The hands are placed flat, side by side on the skin and then moved in a circular fashion, either in the same or in opposite directions. The hands always remain in the same position relative to each other and should not merely slide over the skin. If the area to be massaged is small then the same movements can be performed by the fingertips or with the thumbs. But it is important that full contact is maintained and that the tissues are really moved. It has been said that to do kneading well, the operator should have a good hand with pastry!

Striking

There are two examples of this form of manipulation. One is a specialised technique used to loosen secretions from the chest (as in cystic fibrosis), and which does not form part of this text. The second is a movement designed to increase local circulation and to stimulate the body. The hands are held as though grasping a tennis ball. The elbows are then pushed well away from the body and the hands rotated around the imaginary ball allowing the little finger only to strike the skin. The beat should be fairly quick but light and great care must be taken to prevent the administration of a 'karate chop'. The technique, known as 'hacking' is extremely difficult to do well but is very effective when done efficiently. It is a useful way of ending a massage routine.

There are a number of massage books on the market and they appear to describe and illustrate a wide range of techniques. But they are all, in fact, variations on these three basic themes. Once these have been understood and mastered, they can be changed or varied as the operator wishes.

MASSAGE ROUTINES

Since massage is given to achieve certain defined aims, it is important for it to be ordered and logical. If the aim is to clear localised swelling, then the emphasis should be on stroking to clear the vessels with vigorous kneading to loosen oedema. If relaxation is required, then lighter stroking might well be more appropriate. Routines should be constructed based on what is to be achieved and are therefore variable. However, it is useful to consider a 'model' massage routine as a guideline.

'Model' massage routine

The following sequence is adopted:

(1) Light stroking along the length of the area to be treated — preferably along the lines of the venous drainage.
(2) Kneading to a small proximal area.
(3) Stroking to that area.
(4) Stroking over the entire area along the lines of drainage.
(5) Kneading to an adjacent area.
(6) Stroking over that area.
(7) Stroking over the entire area long the lines of drainage.
(8) Finish with striking for stimulation; deep stroking for relaxation.

It must be emphasised that in therapy the crucial factor is the effect that one wishes to achieve. This to a large extent determines which manipulations are used and whether they are carried out quickly or slowly, deeply or lightly.

The known effects of massage are now summarised in order to make the choice of manipulation or routine easier.

EFFECTS OF MASSAGE

In general terms, massage produces, by the mechanical stimulation of the tissues:

(1) changes in arterial, venous and lymphatic flow.
(2) reflex activity in the central, peripheral and autonomic nervous systems.

Effects of stroking

Given in the direction of venous return, it aids drainage. To make this more effective each stroke should end at the level of the relevant lymph node complex:

(1) in the upper limb, at the bend of the elbow and in the axilla;
(2) in the lower limb, behind the knee and in the groin.

This produces:

(1) increase in drainage;
(2) facilitation of removal of waste products of exercise, fatigue or trauma;
(3) increase in local circulation;
(4) relaxation if done lightly; stimulation if heavily.

Effects of kneading

This produces:

(1) mobilisation of soft tissues;
(2) passive movement of tissue fluids;
(3) increase in circulation.

Effects of striking

This produces:

(1) stimulation of tissues leading to an increase in circulation.

Psychological effects

A personal relationship between therapist and patient in the clinical situation can be established, based on:

(1) touch as a social and therapeutic medium;
(2) the non-verbal communication derived from touch;
(3) the one-to-one ratio with total attention being given to the task in hand.

125

Contraindications to massage

These include:

(1) acute conditions where there is evidence of active inflammation, or in the presence of bleeding or infection;
(2) circulatory problems such as thrombosis, varicose veins, atherosclerosis or arteriosclerosis;
(3) open wounds or skin disease;
(4) following drug therapy (for example, steroids) that might alter the quality of the skin;
(5) loss of skin sensation;
(6) active growths;
(7) psychological aversion to being handled or touched.

MASSAGE IN HEALTH CARE

Massage holds one clear advantage over many other forms of therapy, in that its principles and applications are known and understood by a variety of medical cultures and contexts. Its theoretical basis lies firmly in the physical world and it can be explained in terms of concepts derived from anatomy, biology or psychology. This often makes its use more acceptable to western practitioners used to working within the current mechanical model of practice. The manipulations used in massage are, for the most part, self-explanatory and techniques are easy to understand. No real harm is done if techniques are varied or done in an entirely different way. The application of such techniques produce an obvious mechanical effect that can be readily appreciated and immediate feedback can be obtained about quality or effectiveness. The inter-action during massage allows for the establishment of a positive relationship that can contribute towards an appropriate healing environment.

From the practitioner's point of view, mastery of basic massage techniques produces a degree of manual dexterity that is invaluable in clinical practice. More confidence is gained in the handling of painful parts of the body, and there is a greater sensitivity to the physical and psychological responses that are the manifestations of trauma.

It would be wrong to assert that massage has no disadvantages as a therapy. Its major problem is its unfortunate association with sexual expression, and this has to some extent muted its value as a legitimate therapy within orthodox medicine. Where it has been used it has been formalised to such an extent that it hardly qualifies as an expression of caring. In practical terms, massage is tiring to carry out, and in a number of cases other forms of treatment are as effective while being both quicker and cheaper.

Nevertheless, massage has an important part to play in modern health care. It has great potential for both complementary medicine and for nursing, in that it represents an effective non-technological form of care. Its place in a variety of cultures makes it ideal for reintroduction into indigenous health care particularly in countries that cannot afford to support a medical system based on high technology and expensive drugs. Massage can contribute in a very real way to the awareness and sensitivity of the therapist, making him or her more effective in holistic practice.

CONCLUSIONS

Massage, then, represents a legitimate, non-technological form of therapy that is understood by everyone, largely because its concepts, principles and methods fall within everyday experience. A variety of physical effects can be demonstrated and appreciated. A number of phenomena are also associated with the implications of physical contact and these are important in the life of any individual.

My own practice deals primarily with orthopaedic problems. This involves the management of soft tissue trauma suffered at work, in the home or during sporting activities. While such injuries are clearly associated with changes in the musculo-skeletal structure of the body, they also generate anxiety and the real or imagined threat of disability, prolonged pain, loss of status or employment. Clients have often previously received only 'mechanical' treatment such as surgery, medication or immobilisation; and while these procedures have offered an expedient way of dealing with a particular problem, clients have reported a sense of a lack of care and understanding of their situation. From a purely mechanistic perspective, massage provides a useful way of reaching and affecting the tissues of the body. It would be inaccurate to imply that massage *alone* can provide a universal panacea for disease and ill-health, but it can be employed to great effect as an adjunct to other therapies. I find that the time spent on massage gives the client the time, opportunity and the confidence to share a problem, with the assurance that it will be heard sympathetically without the rush and hurry that characterises many medical interviews. My own manipulation of the tissues imparts a clearer picture of the state of the injured parts and gives a variety of clues about the physical and mental state of the individual. The physical contact represents a sharing of the experience of pain and disability, which in turn, I feel, leads to a sense of empathy and of reassurance and confidence in the therapy provided.

Massage implies a commitment to this approach since it is impossible to wholly separate the social, physical and psychological aspects of touch. If it is done with a real sense of care, then the results far exceed the expectations derived solely from a knowledge of the physiological effects of massage. Above all, massage is a personal therapy in every sense of the word and therefore it must be used with care, discretion and discipline. Nevertheless it represents an effective weapon in the fight to rebuild the damaged integrity of the individual.

REFERENCES

1. LeShan, L. *Holistic Health* (Turnstone Press, London, 1984), Ch. 1.

2. Ilich, I. *Limits to Medicine* (Penguin, Harmondsworth, 1976), p. 11.

3. Wood, E.C. and Becker, P.D. *Beard's Massage* (W.B. Saunders, Philadelphia, 1981), Ch. 4.

4. Tucker, W.E. *Sportsmen and their Injuries* (Pelham Books, London, 1978), pp. 108–12.

5. Fisher, S.V. and Helm, P.A. *Comprehensive Rehabilitation of Burns* (Williams and Wilkins, Baltimore, 1984), pp. 169–70.

6. Gibson, J.J. *The Senses Considered as a Perceptual System* (Allen and Unwin, London, 1966).

7. Frank, L. 'Tactile Communication', *Genetic Psychology Monographs* (1957), 56, pp. 211–55.

8. Montagu, A. *Touching: The Human Significance of the Skin* (Harper and Row, London, 1977).

9. Pratt, J.W. and Mason, A. *The Caring Touch* (Heyden/HM and M, London, 1981), pp. 29–43.

10. Harlow. H.F. and Harlow, M.K. 'Social Deprivation in Monkeys', *Scientific American* (1966), 207, pp. 137–46.

11. Kamenetz, H.L. 'History of Massage', in S. Licht, *Massage, Manipulation and Traction* (E. Licht, Connecticut, 1960).

12. Kleen, E.A.G. *Massage and Medical Gymnastics* (J. and A. Churchill, London, 1918), pp. 6–11.

13. Dicke, E. *Meine Bindesgewebsmassage* (Marquardt, Stuttgart, 1953).

14. Ebner, M. *Connective Tissue Massage* (Robert Krieger, New York, 1980).

USEFUL ADDRESSES

Independent Register of Manipulative Therapists Ltd
106 Crowstone Road
Westcliffe-on-Sea
Essex
SS0 8LQ

The London and Counties Society of Physiologists
100 Waterloo Road
Blackpool
FY4 1AW
Telephone: 0253 403548

9

Yoga

Janet Southall

INTRODUCTION

Yoga is a potent therapy by which anyone can obtain considerable benefit in the prevention and treatment of health disorders.

It promotes the health care of the whole person on each level of his/her existence — physical, psychological, emotional and spiritual. In their definition of 'holistic health' the British Holistic Medical Association[1] also promote each of these areas as contributing towards total health and wellbeing. It is intended for anyone, regardless of condition of health, age, religion or nationality.

Yoga promotes health care not only through self-awareness and personal development, but also attempts to manifest each person's self-healing capacity. In particular it is of considerable benefit in stress-related disorders and in promoting relaxation. In this respect research has demonstrated that people who feel they are continually under stress not only become tired or suffer from anxiety, restlessness, insomnia and so on, but that these can lead to physical manifestations such as hypertension, asthma or gastric ulcers.[2-4] There may also be links between stress and cancers, rheumatic conditions and so on.

With this in mind the practice of yoga can be beneficial to both the health carer and patient as a preventive and remedial therapy. It would seem that both nurses and health care workers are engaged in increasingly stressful work. Growing demands are made upon their time, while problems of understaffing, underfunding and overwork become more apparent daily.

In this stressful context staff cannot hope to provide the optimum physical, emotional and spiritual care required for their patients without depleting their own energy resources or caring adequately for themselves.

Many of these issues can be greatly alleviated by yoga not only in reducing stress and tension, but in promoting greater awareness of our own health needs whether physical, emotional or spiritual. Yoga can be used as a preventive measure, ideally as a way of life, or in conjunction with conventional medical treatment since the practices are gentler, have no side-effects and cater for each person individually according to their needs and capacity.

The aim of this chapter is to outline the origins of yoga and the techniques currently practised today. As will be noted, while the overall aim of yoga is to promote an holistic lifestyle and status of health, there are subtle shifts in technique and emphasis given to certain procedures; thus individuals may choose which style they feel may best suit them. It is helpful to be aware of the range of yoga practices available since many people may assume yoga involves only one technique. Additional information is also given at the end of the chapter concerning the practices of yoga — for example, the Yoga for Health Foundation, a registered charity that has been applying and developing the remedial aspects of yoga for several years.

Yoga is believed to be of Indian origin and to have been devised many thousands of years ago by wise men who understood the nature of man and what was needed for him to live in harmony with himself and the universe. It is now firmly established, as thousands of people are becoming aware of the effectiveness of the techniques in preventing and correcting both physical and emotional problems. Many claims have been made of yoga — for example to retard ageing, promote physical strength and flexibility, enhance looks and posture and develop a sense of purpose and understanding of life.[5]

THE AIMS OF YOGA

Yoga aims to prevent disease by treating the person as a whole, rather than symptoms only. It puts great emphasis on the care and attention to the body, teaches that it is the harmony of the body and mind that determines health; thus when there is disharmony there is disease. Yoga works on the theory that inappropriate mental attitudes cause imbalances and that they are under the control of the patient.[6]

131

The word yoga comes from the ancient Sanskrit language and means union, joining or yoking. It has many levels of interpretation, and one is the uniting together of ourselves physically, mentally, emotionally and spiritually into one harmonious whole. Its ultimate aim is the yoking of our individual self with the universal spirit to attain self-realisation. Individuals are viewed as part of the universe, and as such every aspect of our lives must be taken into account when promoting health.

HISTORY

The origins of yoga are obscure and uncertain because dates and exact authorship of many writings were never written down.

Gnana yoga

Excavations that were carried out in the Indus valley of North-east India around 1920 indicate that yoga was already in existence in about 2500–1500 BC.[7] Stone seals were unearthed depicting figures in the meditative sitting postures of yoga revealing that the yoga being practised then was introspective and contemplative. This is known as Gnana yoga — the yoga of wisdom and knowledge. It is concerned with using the mind to study and enquire into one's own nature. It teaches that our minds and bodies should be viewed as part of a continuum and not as separate entities seemingly unrelated to one another. In this way Gnana yoga advocates that one can gain a clearer understanding of life, of our place in the universe, and also an experience of the 'truth'.

It is believed these contemplatives or Gnani yogis obtained great insight into the nature of man, the universe and of man's need to come into harmony with himself and the universe. These were handed down by word of mouth over a period of many centuries from master to disciple and from generation to generation in the form of chants, rituals and poetry which showed the development of yoga from early Indian spiritual thoughts to the abstract concept of the Absolute Brahman.

Later, these were written down in the four Vedas which are considered to be the oldest books of spiritual writing in the world (the word 'Veda' means knowledge). The later writings of the Vedas formed the Upanishads[7] which literally mean 'sitting at the feet of the Master for instruction'. Many Upanishads were written down and collected over a long period of time — of these ten were chosen as being unique and of lasting value and all have now been translated.

Raja yoga

About 300 BC the teachings were collected and codified by an Indian scholar,[7] Patanjali, in the writing known as the Yoga Sutras of Patanjali. This is a book of instruction giving a code of ethics and an explanation of Raja yoga. The name is derived from the fact that it enables one to become king or raja over one's inner powers. Sutra means 'thread' which implies that there is an underlying continuous thought throughout the writings. The human mind is explored and strict definite guidelines are laid down for its control. The nature of enlightenment is discussed, the means by which it is attained — the obstacles — problems of practice and ways of overcoming them. Patanjali states that the mind has a great influence on the physical body, and also that the main psychological hindrance to self-realisation is ignorance of the true nature of reality.

Bhagavad Gita

About the same time as Patanjali was formulating the Sutras the *Bhagavad Gita* (song of the Lord) was composed.[7] As with all the writings it was written in Sanskrit, the ancient Indian language, but the author is unknown. This offers a way of life for everyone in all walks of life to follow, for greater happiness and peace of mind. As with all the teachings they are as applicable today as when they were written.

It describes the pathways of Gnana yoga and Raja yoga but also Karma yoga and Bhakti yoga. These types of yoga overlap but they do not conflict with or oppose each other. They were formed as it was apparent that people were not alike — that backgrounds and individual natures varied and therefore the way that would suit one person would not suit another. Each one of us is different in our approach to life. All paths though lead ultimately to self-improvement and self-realisation.

Karma yoga

Karma yoga is the yoga of doing work that is selfless and without looking for reward. The Sanskrit word 'Karma' interprets into the Law of Cause and Effect. Every effect has a cause so it follows that good generates good and evil generates evil. Karma yoga teaches us how to avoid future troubles by our conduct now and in our approach to every thought, word and deed.

Bhakti yoga

Bhakti yoga is the yoga of love and devotion. It is followed by those who think with the heart and not the head, for the people who live by emotion rather than intellect. It is not necessarily a devotion to religion. It can be a daily devotion in everyday activities, as in a mother devoted to her home and family.

'Aids' to yoga — Mantra yoga and Yantra yoga

These were developed at a later date as aids to meditation and took the form of the repetition of certain sounds and words, which is Mantra yoga, and the use of geometric designs, which is Yantra yoga.

Patanjali's eight limbs

All yoga teaching is based on Patanjali's eight limbs or stages which are listed and explained in part of the second and third chapters of his writings (Ashtanga yoga). They are progressive and interrelated aspects of yoga practice, and as one practises it becomes apparent that the stages cannot be separated. They are the five Yamas and Niyamas — Asana, Pranayama, Pratyahara, Dharana, Dhyana and Samadhi (Table 9.1).

HATHA YOGA AND ITS TECHNIQUES

Hatha yoga is the most widely known and often misunderstood form of yoga. Traditionally the practice of Hatha yoga is a preparation for

Table 9.1: Patanjali's eight limbs or stages of yoga called collectively Ashtanga yoga

Yamas	Self-restraints, moral prohibitions, social interactions or duties to others.
Niyamas	Self-discipline and observances.

To practice the Yamas and Niyamas progressively, allowing them to enter more and more into everyday activities is a step towards self-healing.

Asana	A posture that is meant for mediation.
Pranayama	Prana means breath — Ayama is lengthening through control. Breathing is controlled.
Pratyahara	The withdrawing of the senses inward away from outside stimuli — detracting the senses from the mind in preparation for the next step.
Dharana	Concentration and confinement of the mind to one point, object or area.
Dhyana	Meditation, contemplation.
Samadhi	Spiritual or superconsciousness.

Raja yoga. The classical text is the Hatha Yoga Pradipika which means 'the light with which to see yoga', and was compiled by a sage called Swatmarama in about 1600 AD. It consists of the same eight limbs as Patanjali's Ashtanga yoga but pays more attention to techniques such as Kriyas — internal cleaning of the body; Asanas — body positions, and Pranayama — breathing exercises.

The word Hatha (pronounced Hat-ha) means balance or force. It is really two words combined. Ha means the sun, positive, expressive, will, energy, and Tha the moon, negative, sense, energy — which are the two opposing currents in the universe. Hatha yoga is the path of energy balance — to balance the sun/moon energies for wholeness and health.

The Kriyas — internal cleanings

These are used to cleanse the nasal passages, the eyes and the respiratory and digestive tracts. Traditionally there are six techniques. Some of them may seem bizarre to the westerner, but some can actually be adapted for our use (Table 9.2).

Table 9.2: Internal cleansings of the body*

Title	Aim and benefit	Procedure
1. Kapalabhati (shining skull)	Clears the mind Aids concentration Beneficial for helping to clear a cold	Breathing exercise: The breath is exhaled forcefully and inhaled passively a number of times followed by a few deep breaths.
2. Neti	Cleanses the nasal passages	The introduction of plain water into the nostrils alternately by the use of a small spouted pot, the water running out of the mouth or by the passing of a catheter into the nose and out through the mouth.
3. Dhauti	The cleansing of the stomach	The swallowing and withdrawing of a bandage. A western alternative could be the drinking of hot water and lemon on rising, also fasting.
4. Basti	The cleansing of the colon and intestines	The technique is to squat in a tub of water and to draw up the water through a tube inserted into the anus by the strong abdominal movement of Uddiyana and Nauli which creates a natural vacuum. A western version would be an enema.
5. Uddiyana Bandha and Nauli	Beneficial effect on the internal organs and intestinal upsets	The abdominal muscles are drawn upwards and contracted in Uddiyana Bandha as a preparation for Nauli in which the abdominal recti muscles are isolated and moved in a churning action.
6. Trataka	The cleansing of the eyes	An object is gazed at until the eyes begin to water.

*Such techniques should not be attempted unless with a competent practitioner.

The Asanas — body positions

Pronounced Ars-na, the word comes from the Sanskrit root meaning 'to sit', and traditionally it means holding a posture or pose firmly and effortlessly so that the mind is freed to practise meditation. There are alleged to be many thousands of different postures but it is believed that 84 is the classical number. These are the techniques with which most people in the West are familiar, and form a thorough complete exercise system working on all aspects of existence.

Asanas are powerful, efficient and effective as they are scientific patterns of posture designed to work on all areas of the body so that the whole body can benefit. Each one. is designed to work on a *specific* area of the body.

The effect of the Asanas

They act therapeutically by physiologically appearing to help all parts of the body to work with maximum efficiency. The endocrine system is stimulated so that the glands work more efficiently. The internal viscera are also stimulated for increased efficiency. The muscles and joints are exercised correctly, so progressively the range of movement can increase, keeping the joints mobile and healthy. The circulation is improved and this in turn affects the whole of the body. With the inverted postures the veins in the legs are affected, putting the feet up being one treatment for varicose veins; they act as postural drainage and are considered antiageing as they reverse the pull of gravity.[3]

They act psychologically by developing an inner calm, overcoming tension and disciplining the mind so that it is able to concentrate; and spiritually by instilling confidence and a greater awareness of life.[9]

Basic breathing and Pranayama

The breathing practices in yoga are divided into two: normal physiological breathing pattern, and the practice of Pranayama.

Most people breathe in a very limited way, not fully using the lungs, and only taking in a reduced amount of oxygen; this results in the body becoming sluggish and the heart being put under strain, leading to illness and upset. This may be due to bad posture, lack of exercise and mental and emotional upsets. When there is worry, fear and tension the breathing is often slow, shallow and jerky, and when there is emotional upset and stress the breath is quick.

Yoga teaches deep breathing by the practice of specific postures which open the chest and stretch the spine, work on the diaphragm and other muscles involved in breathing, and also by basic breathing exercises. These are carefully graded to open up, progressively, all areas of the lungs such as with diaphragmatic, thoracic and clavicular breathing techniques.

Pranayama is the control of vital energy through the breath — Ayama means 'control' and Prana is vital energy or life force, which is all-pervading and is the sum total of cosmic energy. It is said to be present in air, food, sunshine and water although it has never been isolated as one of their constituents. Prana is taken into the body in all of these but chiefly in air. The effects of Prana are believed to be healing and the more the body is permeated with Pranic energy the less likely it is to become diseased.

Pranayama techniques put specific emphasis on a prolonged exhalation and holding the breath both out and in. The prolonged exhalation appears to have a tranquillising effect that can be helpful to many students and people who are emotionally upset. The retention of the breath out slows the breathing down generally and also the heart rate, while the retention of the breath in stimulates cellular breathing.[10] By concentrating on breathing in this way the mind acts as the bridge between body and mind, between the conscious mind and subconscious psyche. It is not advisable for anyone with a heart upset or detached retina to hold the breath out or in.

Traditionally, Pranayama exercises are performed while sitting in one of the classical sitting postures with the head, neck and spine in a straight line to allow for the expansion of the chest and for the mind to be able to concentrate but they can be performed sitting in a chair, a wheelchair or lying down, for example while in bed. Of the eight Pranayamas listed in the classical texts the technique of alternate nostril breathing is immensely beneficial for its tranquillising effect. This is performed by closing one nostril alternatively with the fingers and using the other nostril.

RELAXATION

This is an important and essential part of all yoga sessions. It helps one to obtain benefit from the practice but can also be a valuable daily practice for both nurses and patients alike. So often stress is the result of being unable to relax and it is believed that more disease is caused by stress than any other factor.[3]

Relaxation is interpreted as a re-creation of the energy in the body and should not be confused with recreation in which one is actively involved in an enjoyable pastime or the view that relaxation is sprawling in a chair. It is time of 'not doing', of letting go in order to release muscular tension, recharge the batteries, and for mental calmness. It is having the correct amount of contraction and relaxation in the body to allow the flow of energy. It teaches us how to identify areas of tension in our everyday activities and how to deal with them. This can be of immense value to health care workers who may be working in areas of high patient dependency but with minimal and overstretched staffing resources. It is said that its practice will help one deal with difficult situations and upheavals, and have a profound effect in the prevention and treatment of high blood pressure and its related diseases of heart attacks and strokes.[3]

The yoga way of relaxation is easy to learn. There are three stages:

(1) Physical relaxation which involves the tensing and relaxing of each part of the body in turn from the tips of the toes to the top of the head.
(2) Mental relaxation — watching the breath as the breath is allowed to flow naturally and letting go of all thoughts, worries, fears, distractions.
(3) Spiritual relaxation — here relaxation is allowed to develop so as to experience an inner peace and calm.

There are many variations of this sequence. For the practice to be rewarding it is important that one does not try to relax or to look for relaxation as this will actually prevent it. At the end of the time, which may be from 5 to 15 minutes, great care must be taken to bring the consciousness into the body before moving. The posture is preferably one of lying down on the floor but the sequence may also be performed lying in a bed.

MEDITATION IN YOGA

There are two types of meditation: passive, involving the actual practice of meditation; and active, which can occur spontaneously during everyday activities no matter how mundane, menial or involved. Meditation is described in the last four stages or steps of Patanjali's Yoga Sutras as:

(1) Pratyahara: sense withdrawal.
(2) Dharana: concentration.
(3) Dhyana: meditation.
(4) Samadhi: superconsciousness.

Pratyahara

Pratyahara is the checking and curbing of the outward tendencies of the mind so that awareness can be directed within. It involves bringing the senses under control. This can be practised as an exercise, or it can become a natural progression of the practice of the previous Sutras, Pratyahara being the preparation for the last three steps known collectively as Samyana.

Dharana

Dharana is concerned with fixing the mind on one object to the exclusion of all else. The object should be something that suits the nature and personality of the person and so absorbing that one becomes completely lost in it, for example, a flower, fruit or the recitation of a word or phrase (as in Mantra yoga).

Dhyana and Samadhi

Dhyana is the state into which one will automatically fall, leading to Samadhi which is the experience of peace, when true knowledge becomes a reality.

Research on meditation

Meditation has been carefully and scientifically examined.[3] It has been discovered that the oxygen intake is reduced by about 20 per cent during this state against the 5 per cent of the person who flops into a chair, even though in each case the body is physically inactive.[3] The brain consumes the largest amount of oxygen in the body and a lowering of consumption shows that there is reduced brain activity; the latter is mainly involved with the uncontrolled thoughts we all have. Consequently this uses up a large amount of natural energy, leaving us exhausted and depleted and liable to disease.

It has also been discovered in meditation that at the same time as there is a decrease in the respiratory rate there is an increase in skin resistance and alpha-wave activity.[3] This means a decrease in activity of the sympathetic nervous system, and an increase in the activity of the parasympathetic nervous system.

It is obvious that there is a great deal of overlap between relaxation and meditation in its beginning stages.[11] The quietening down of the sympathetic nervous system is similar in both these techniques.[12] In fact in terms of physiology deep relaxation produces the same alteration in skin resistance, brain waves and breath patterns as meditation.[13]

A recent survey of the world medical and scientific literature on meditation and other self-control strategies came to the conclusion that various kinds of meditation, relaxation methods, yoga and biofeedback were equivalent from the point of view of health benefits.[14]

DIET IN YOGA

> Yoga is a harmony. Not for him who eats too much or for him who eats too little.
>
> *Bhagavad Gita*[15]

Yoga teaches that there is a close relationship between the kind of foods we eat and the body, mind and emotions, and puts food into three categories. Sattvic for purity, Rajasic for activity, and Tamasic for inertia, which are the Gunas or inherent qualities of nature. These qualities coexist in equilibrium in all things, although one will always be dominant.

Sattvic foods

Sattvic foods are natural, pure and completely unadulterated, and include fruit, vegetables, grains, wholemeal bread, nuts, seeds, honey, herb teas and whole foods. These help to encourage the body to become healthy, the mind clear and alert, and discourage disease.

Rajasic and Tamasic foods

The Rajasic and Tamasic foods are not pure, wholesome or fresh; they have a dulling effect on the mind and make the body lethargic, as large amounts of natural energy are required to digest and metabolise the food.

Traditionally a yogic diet excludes meat. This is primarily because of the ethical principle that it is wrong to kill an animal as all life is sacred. The protein found in meat can be replaced by nuts and dairy produce, and by combining certain foods to ensure a healthy balanced diet. A vegetarian eats a Sattvic diet. As yoga practice develops so will the desire to change one's eating habits. It is important, though, for any change to be gradual and for a diet to be correctly balanced.

YOGA TODAY

A basic yoga session

A basic yoga session may vary in length from 1 to 2 hours; it may contain a large or small number of students, or a session can be on a one-to-one basis. The venue can be, for example, in a centre administered by an adult education service, or in a community day centre organised by a social services department, or it can be organised privately by the teacher, perhaps in the day room of a hospital ward or even in the home of the student.

A session would start with a period of centring in the relaxation posture as a physical and mental preparation in order to become composed to derive all possible benefit from the practice.

The postures are then practised after a period of limbering up designed to loosen and warm the body. They are planned to move the body completely and safely either in a dynamic or static way or a combination of both. The use of counter posture — that is, if the spine has been bent one way then the next posture would bend it the opposite way — and relaxation practices ensure that the posture session is perfectly balanced. It is important that the student works without strain or force and without competition.

All postures can be modified and altered for any student who is restricted in any way, perhaps due to being elderly or unwell, for example by sitting in a chair, a wheelchair or by using straps and cushions to help with the 'feel' of a posture. The accompanying illustrations (Figures 9.1, 9.2 and 9.3) show a selection of basic postures and how a chair can be used by anyone who has difficulty in standing.

Postures can also be 'graded' and used according to the capacity of the class or individual; for example they can be strenuous and demanding for the fit (Figures 9.4 and 9.5) or gently used for those who may be ill (Figure 9.6).

Everyone can derive immense benefit from a practice, however fit or unwell that person is, and no one should feel disheartened.

Figure 9.1: A side bending posture

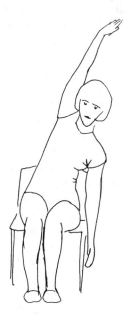

Figure 9.2: A forward bending posture

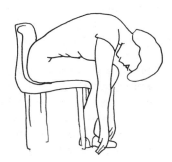

After the posture session breathing exercises are taught and the practice is completed by a period of relaxation. There may also be a meditation session and a talk, and discussion on a philosophical aspect of yoga or other topics depending on the experience and capacity of the student. No special equipment is required to practise yoga — just a mat, rug or large towel for use on the floor and loose-fitting clothing that does not restrict movement and stretching.

As postures can be modified and altered to suit a student so can a whole session or class. Such are remedial classes that would emphasise centring, slowing and lengthening the breath, limbering and stretching for a few basic postures and breathing exercises and could be useful in helping recovery and a feeling of wellbeing.

CONCLUSIONS: YOGA IN NURSING AND HEALTH CARE PRACTICE

These teachings comprise a holistic approach to health care. There is little in the teachings to cause conflict with anyone or anything as they are all natural and in tune with nature and the laws of the universe. This approach is of vital importance in our stress-ridden society.

Most people become interested in yoga as a means of improving

Figure 9.3: A backward bending posture

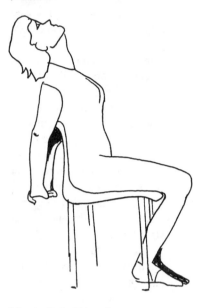

Figure 9.4: Triangle pose

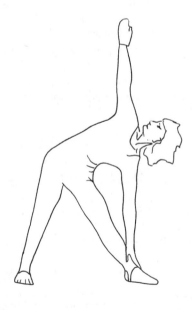

physical fitness, to reduce discomforts and to help in relieving specific ailments such as arthritis, high blood pressure, respiratory conditions, back pain, multiple sclerosis and many other upsets. Others are becoming interested in yoga as a natural way of releasing tension and stress by learning and practising the relaxation techniques; and some are looking for help and guidance in living life more fully.

Whatever the reason for the interest in yoga it becomes progressively a way of life. Once learnt from a teacher many of the techniques can be adapted and used during everyday activities wherever one happens to be and can be done very unobtrusively to help one to cope, to be relaxed and balanced whatever the situation. They need only take a few minutes at odd times, such as having a 2 minute break in the form of a quiet time, meditatively with the eyes closed observing the breath or doing a breathing exercise. Also being aware of posture, and correcting it if necessary, guards against building up pockets of tension and promotes a feeling of peace and wellbeing in addition to an awareness of thoughts, attitudes and expressions, developing positivity.

Figure 9.5: A forward bending pose

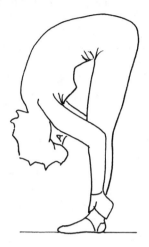

Figure 9.6: Relaxation position: modified

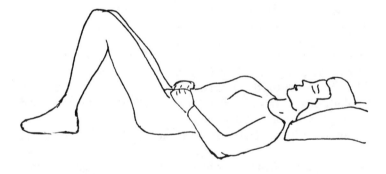

Yoga then becomes a self-help therapy from which we can learn that each and everyone of us is responsible for our own health. Nurses and health care workers can use yoga for their own benefit, health and wellbeing and can safely recommend it to their patients either by helping them personally, by learning the techniques, or advising them to contact a yoga teacher for instruction. Lists can be obtained from all the organisations listed under 'Additional Information'.

Yoga is a powerful therapeutic tool for self-development and self-discovery which benefits the individual, society and the world. We

145

can experience a greater harmony with ourselves and the world by following well thought-out principles and practising them consistently.

ADDITIONAL INFORMATION

At the present time research into yoga is taking place both in India and the West.

The British Wheel of Yoga is a registered charity, founded in 1963, whose purpose is to help all persons to a greater knowledge and understanding of all aspects of yoga and its practice by the provision of facilities for research, study, education and training and which desires to co-operate with and support other organisations having similar objectives. (Constitution 1979).

Further information and details of yoga classes and teachers can be obtained from Dr Kendall, General Secretary, Grafton Grange, Grafton, North Yorkshire.

The Yoga for Health Foundation is a registered charity which runs a residential centre and has been cultivating the remedial aspects of yoga for many years. It also provides training schemes, seminars and visits for the well and sick. For some time the Yoga for Health Foundation has been applying yoga techniques to multiple sclerosis with distinctly favourable results. Write to Ickwell Bury, Northill, Biggleswade, Bedfordshire for additional information and details of their yoga classes and teachers.

Yoga Biomedical Trust researches into the therapeutic effects of yoga as a means of improving the mental, physical and spiritual health of the community. For further information contact Dr Robin Monro, PO Box 140, Cambridge, CB1 1PU.

REFERENCES

1. British Holistic Medical Asociation, *What is Holistic Medicine?* (British Holistic Medical Association, London, 1985).
2. Assagioli, R. *The Act of Will* (Penguin, Baltimore, Maryland, 1974).
3. Benson, H. *The Relaxation Response*, 3rd impression (Collins Fount Paperbacks, London, 1982).
4. Brena, S.F. *Yoga and Medicine* (Penguin, Harmondsworth, 1973).

5. Reiker, H.U. *The Yoga of Light* (George Allen and Unwin, London, 1972).

6. Garde, R.K. *Principles and Practice of Yoga Therapy* (Wolfe Publishing Ltd, London, 1975).

7. Worthington, V. *A History of Yoga* (Routledge and Kegan Paul Ltd, London, 1982).

8. Chandra, F. *Medical and Physiological Aspects of Yoga* (University Yoga Publications, Connington, Cambridge, 1979).

9. Bhole, M.V. *Therapeutic Importance of Yoga Practices* (University Yoga Publications, Connington, Cambridge, 1974).

10. Van Lysbeth, A. *Pranayama* (Unwin Paperbacks, London, 1979).

11. Huxley, A.L. *The Art of Seeing* (Montana Books, Seattle, Washington, 1974).

12. Kamiya, J. *Biofeedback and Self-control* (Aldine, Atherton, Chicago, 1971).

13. James, G., Dennis, J. and Bresler, D. (eds) *Mind, Body and Health: Towards an Integral Medicine* (National Institute of Mental Health, Rockwill, Maryland, 1981).

14. Lamb, W. and Watson, E. *Body Code — The Meaning in Movement* (Routledge and Kegan Paul Ltd, London, 1982).

15. Radice, B. and Baldick, R. (eds) *Bhagavad Gita*, Chapter 6, Volume 16, p. 70. Penguin Classics, translated by Juan Mascaro (Penguin, Harmondsworth).

BIBLIOGRAPHY AND FURTHER READING

Many books have now been written about yoga. They can be obtained from Angela's Yoga Books, 65 Norfolk Road, Seven Kings, Ilford, Essex. A list will be supplied upon application.

The Bhagavad Gita (Pengiun Classics, Harmondsworth, 1st edn 1962).

Brosnan, B. *Yoga for Handicapped People* (Souvenir Press, London, 1982).

Kent, H. *Yoga for the Disabled* (Thorsons, Wellingborough, 1985).

Reiker, H.U. *The Hatha Yoga Pradipika* (George Allen and Unwin, London, 1972).

Sivananda Yoga Centre *The Book of Yoga* (Ebury Press, London, 1983).

Taimni, I.K. *Science of Yoga* (Quest Books, Theosophical Publishing House, Wheaton, Illinois, 1961).

The Upanishads (Penguin Classics, Harmondsworth, 1st edn 1965).

Wood, E. *Yoga* (Pengiun Books, Harmondsworth, 1982).

Worthington, V. *A History of Yoga* (Routledge and Kegan Paul Ltd, London, 1982).

10

Healing: Therapeutic Touch

Pat Turton

INTRODUCTION

'Laying on of hands', whether it is called faith healing or therapeutic touch, is arguably one of the most sought-after of the complementary therapies. In Holland in 1980 for example, 6.5 per cent of the total population had visited a healer.[1] It would seem reasonable to assume that an equally large number of British people have recourse to this form of therapy with 20 000 healers practising in the United Kingdom.[2] Unfortunately, however, there are no published figures to substantiate this claim.

What is clear is that for many people visiting a healer is not an obvious step but an act of desperation when scientific medicine appears to have no more to offer them.[3] In one study almost three-quarters of the people who consulted a healer did so because of the failure of medical or other therapies. Nor were their hopes disappointed. Of the 116 respondents, 30 per cent made a complete recovery, 25 per cent a partial recovery, and 24 per cent an improved ability to cope with symptoms.[4] It would be simplistic, however, to equate successful healing with the cure of illness — there is also what may be called 'inner healing', which is particularly relevant in support of the terminally ill, for example.

Healing may relieve disease by enhancing the client/patient self-coping mechanism, for example, reducing anxiety, increasing self-esteem, though it may not shrink the tumour or make the blind see.

HISTORY AND DEVELOPMENT OF THERAPY

When a mother places her hand on her child's fevered brow and wishes him better, she is healing — and as such healing by laying on of hands is probably as old as the human race.

In his book *The Power to Heal*, David Harvey[4] traces the written history of healing back 5,000 years to the ancient texts of China and India. Both these civilisations recognised the existence of an 'energy' or force that could be channelled for the benefit of the sick person. In China it was called Qi and in India Prana.

In the West, according to Harvey, healing was first documented by the Greek cult of Aesculapius. And 500 years later, in the fifth century BC, Hippocrates the father of modern medicine was noted for his healing gift of 'laying on of hands'.

The most famous healer in western tradition is Jesus Christ and the New Testament testifies to the numerous and spectacular cures he performed. The Church continued this healing ministry, though it is no longer as dominant a feature of church activity as it was in the first few hundred years of its foundation.

With the rise of Christianity, healing was claimed as the exclusive domain of the clergy. Anyone who practised healing without sanction of the Church was liable to be prosecuted under the anti-witchcraft laws. Despite this injunction, however, many individuals other than priests continued to practise this form of healing. One of the most famous of the lay healers described by Harvey[4] was a Puritan called Valentine Greatrakes, whose gift for curing diseases was in great demand. Contemporary accounts of his work during 1665 claim 'above three score cured by him in one night of deafness, blindness, cancers, sciatica, palsies, impostumes, fistulas and the like, who went away by the blessing of God well recovered' (p. 143).[4]

Despite an ecclesiastical injunction forbidding him to do so Greatrakes, probably because of his high social standing, continued to heal and no further action was taken against him. Indeed he is noteworthy as one of the first healers to have encouraged scientific scrutiny of his work by members of the Royal Society such as the chemist, Boyle. In the same period, however, many were executed as witches for practising the same healing gift as Greatrakes. This uneasy and often hostile relationship between the established churches and the lay healers has continued — though with less dire consequences for the healers — until the present day.

Indeed as one English healer, Bruce MacManaway says 'Until as late as 1951, I and others like me ran the theoretical risk of arrest under the Witchcraft Act which carried the death penalty, even if it had not been used for some time' (p. 24).[5]

In the 1950s MacManaway was himself involved in two important commissions on healing: one by the Bishops of Canterbury and York (1958), and the other by the British Medical Association (1956). Neither commission, according to MacManaway, actually referred to the evidence. The cases presented by the healers were not considered, yet both commissions 'concluded that any cure that is claimed to have resulted from healing is in fact due to wrong diagnosis, wrong prognosis, suggestion, remission or spontaneous healing' (p. 29)[5] though as MacManaway points out 'The latter two explanations are surely only ways of saying that something has happened but no one knows why' (p. 29).[5]

But despite the negative conclusions of both commissions, public interest in healing has been increasingly positive since the 1950s. The National Federation of Spiritual Healers was started in 1955 under the Presidency of the famous healer Harry Edwards, and for the first time healers were able to act as an effective pressure group for change. In 1959, for example, the Federation 'was able to obtain permission from the management committees responsible for over 1500 hospitals to allow accredited healer members of the National Federation of Spiritual Healers into its wards to treat patients' (p. 73).[4]

Traditionally the medical profession, like the Church, has held a negative or dismissive view of healing which was given 'legal' standing by the ban on cooperation between doctors and unqualified healers. In 1977, however, bowing to public opinion the General Medical Council changed its policy and allowed doctors to suggest or agree to their patients seeking the assistance of a healer (p.74).[4] However, by the 1980s, even within the medical profession's own ranks attitudes were changing. A small study in 1983 showed 'a striking degree of interest in alternative methods of treatment among younger doctors'.[6] Healing was one of the therapies considered in the study; over half of the group expressed an opinion with two to one saying that it was useful.[6]

In 1983 too the British Medical Association Board of Science and Education set up an enquiry into the value of alternative therapies.[7] Commenting on healing, the report states that the 'techniques of the faith healers, divine healers and others in associated groups are safe and non-invasive and offer the prospect of increased well-being for many sufferers . . . but we do not believe these methods are of therapeutic value in themselves' (p. 70).[7] Concluding, the British Medical Association report accepted that western medicine has been 'assisted' in the past by concepts and techniques originally from unorthodox sources (p. 78).[7] To be accepted by the medical establishment, however, such therapies, healing among them, must according to the British Medical Association be scientifically validated.

The British Confederation of Healing Organisations, recognising that without such scientific evidence healing will remain outside mainstream health care, set up the Healing Research Project in 1986. It is hoped that the results, if positive, will persuade the British Medical Association and its membership of the value of healing in a language they understand, and there will be further cooperation between health workers and healers within the National Health Service to the benefit of the patients.

HEALING AND CHRISTIANITY

Many western peoples' attitudes and beliefs about healing have been shaped by both the Christian Church and science. The former, while recognising the existence of the healing phenomenon, maintains it to be a direct gift of the Holy Spirit through the intercession of individuals sanctioned by the Church. Healers outside the Church's ambit and control were until recently thought to be heretics in league with demons and spirits and therefore to be condemned. With the 'charismatic renewal' that is current in much of the Christian world, healing, long at the fringes of the Church ministry is once again becoming a major focus.

One of the first Catholics involved in this charismatic renewal, Father Francis MacNutt,[8] maintains that there are three sources of healing power:

1. divine power of God;
2. demonic power from spiritualist sources;
3. a natural force of healing, based on love, which is given to some people.

MacNutt expalins that

> There is some evidence . . . that people with a strong life energy are able to transmit some of this to other people through the laying on of hands. If this is shown to be true I see no reason to fear it any more than any other natural force that we discover, for it ultimately reflects glory to God, its creator (p. 285).[8]

151

This, if it represents the view of many churchmen and church-women, is a very important statement. It allows that healing by other than Christians can provide a morally acceptable adjunct to medical practice. Healing is no longer therefore perceived as either good, that is, when it is done in the name of Jesus, or evil when it is not.

The recognition that healing, as for example a nursing or medical technique, is a natural gift, absolves both the practitioner and receiver from any guilty fear that they may be meddling in superstitious practices. It is worth reiterating the point by quoting MacManaway, who as a committed Christian wrote 'while the Spiritual, God-given aspects of the healing gift is to me very important, healing can nevertheless be viewed on its own as a natural phenomenon' (p. 26).[5]

BASIC ASSUMPTION STUDIES OF HEALING

One of the best-known British healers, explaining his method of healing, wrote: 'I should say that communication between healer and patient sets up an interplay of energy which accelerates the patient's own internal healing'. MacManaway's description postulates two essential processes at work in the act of healing: the *vis medicatrix naturae*, or the healing power of nature, which according to Dr Ian Pearce (p. 15)[9] 'has been largely forgotten by modern medicine'; the energy (Prana/Qi) that accelerates or triggers this self-healing mechanism. The British Medical Association Report,[7] commenting on this concept of energy, wrote:

> In our view, reliance on descriptions of energy flows to account for the effect of alternative therapies, in the absence of precise definitions or an explicit (let alone systematic) theoretical framework, is no more than dogmatic metaphysics . . . We understand the appeal of such concepts to those who wish to reject what they see as the materialism of scientific medicine, but we do not believe that these methods are of therapeutic value in themselves (p. 70).

The scepticism of the British Medical Association reflects the generally held view of doctors that healing is an illusion. As Pearce points out 'despite the growing body of experimental evidence now accumulating that there are powers of healing in certain individuals, which do not fit into the accepted scientific model, medical opinion prefers to ignore the evidence and to dismiss the whole subject as phantasy and wishful thinking' (p. 262).[9]

Examples of the 'experimental evidence' described in detail by Dr Pearce[9] were provided by two biochemists, Dr Bernard Grad and Sister Justa Smith. These scientists worked with a Hungarian healer, Colonel Estabany, during the 1960s at McGill University in Montreal, Canada, and Rosary Hill College, Buffalo, United States. Grad argued that if healing was the result of some force or energy rather than the power of suggestion then it would have observable effects on animals and plants.

He chose, therefore, to test the effect of healing on the rate of wound healing in mice and on the growth of barley seeds. From the series of four controlled experiments (two of which were carried out under double-blind conditions), Grad concluded that the healing of skin wounds in mice was definitely and significantly accelerated in those animals which had been held by the healer.

A comparable effect was found in the experiments on barley seeds, in that 'the treated plants were significantly higher on all days of measurement and that the yield of plant material from the treated group was significantly higher' (p. 267).[9]

Justa Smith chose to examine whether or not healing would positively effect the enzyme trypsin in solution. She found that the samples of solution 'treated' by Estabany showed a significant increase in activity over the control solution.

On the basis of these experiments, Pearce wrote, 'one is forced to conclude, however reluctantly, that there are some people who are able at certain times to generate a form of energy which is capable of interacting with matter and which, for the present, we have no means of instrumenting' (p. 273).[9]

Apart from his work with Grad and Justa Smith, Colonel Estabany acted as healer in three experimental studies undertaken by Dolores Krieger, with haemoglobin as the variable. Using a classic experimental research design they repeatedly confirmed Krieger's hypothesis that

the mean haemoglobin values of the experimental group after treatment by the laying on of hands would exceed their before treatment haemoglobin values, and that the mean haemoglobin values of the control group at comparable times would show no significant difference (confirmed at 0.01 level of confidence in two studies and $p > 0.001$ in another).[10]

It was clear to Krieger from her own and others' research that a 'known' healer could effect accelerated repair in living organisms. What was not established was whether this was a 'special gift'. Krieger herself learnt the technique of laying on of hands and found that she 'could elicit reactions in healees similar to those stated in the literature' (p. 142).[11] In 1974 she tested her assumption that healing was a natural human potential which could be activated by those who had a fairly healthy body (so that they had an over-abundance of Prana energy), a strong intention to help or heal ill persons, and who were educable.[12] The research hypothesis and design was essentially the same as in the haemoglobin studies with Estabany. This study, however, used 32 registered nurses who had been taught healing. The results confirmed the hypothesis (at 0.001 level of confidence),[12] and clearly demonstrated that 'ordinary' nurses were able to produce similar effects, at least on haemoglobin values, as 'known healers'.

Encouraged by these results Dolores Krieger has pioneered the use of healing, or therapeutic touch as she came to call it, as a nursing 'modality'. It is now widely taught in the United States and Canada and practised by nurses 'as a natural extension of their professional skills' (p. 146).[11]

Like MacManaway, Krieger is convinced that the healing involves some form of energy/Prana. The healer, Krieger believes, is an individual whose health gives him/her access to an abundance of this energy and whose strong sense of commitment gives the ability to project this vital energy to supplement the deficit of energy of the patient. On the physical level, Krieger supposes, this occurs by electron resonance. 'The resonance acts in the service of the ill person to re-establish the vitality of the flow in this open system, to restore, as it were unimpeded communication with the environment — for given this, all literature agrees, the patient really heals himself.'[12]

Healing, for Dolores Krieger, is not associated with any specific religious belief or divine intervention. Like the appreciation of music and the playing of an instrument, healing is a gift available to all of us to some extent at least, and which can be developed through training and practice.

WHAT THE THERAPY INVOLVES AND ITS USE IN NURSING

Hippocrates is said by Harvey (p. 34)[4] to offer one of the earliest accounts of the actual process of healing,

> it is believed by experienced doctors that the heat which oozes
> out of the hand, on being applied to the sick, is highly salutory
> . . . It has often appeared while I have been soothing my patients,
> as if there was a singular property in my hands to pull and draw
> away from the affected parts aches and diverse impurities, by laying
> my hand upon the place and by extending my fingers towards it.

Laying on of hands healing, as Dolores Krieger points out, 'looks absurdly simple but is profoundly complex. The act consists of the simple placing of the hands for about 10–15 minutes on or close to the body of an ill person by someone who intends to help or to heal that person'.[10]

Unlike the majority of other healers, Krieger has developed and taught a systematic approach to this 'absurdly simple act'. It is perhaps that, along with her encouragement to research into its mode of action and value within the clinical nursing setting, that distinguishes Krieger's therapeutic touch from other forms of this healing therapy. There are four components or phases to the process of therapeutic touch as outlined by Krieger: centring, assessment, mobilising the energy field, and finally the healer's conscious directing of energy to assist the patient.

Centring

Centring oneself physically and psychologically is finding within oneself an inner reference of stability (p. 35).[13] This is the first and fundamental phase of healing. Essentially the healer must maintain a meditative state throughout the act of healing. The techniques by which this meditative state may be acquired are numerous and well documented (for example, in Meg Bond's book, *Stress and Self Awareness*[14]). Meditation, like any skill, must be practised, but once acquired it becomes possible for the meditative state to be achieved very swiftly and enables the 'healer' to remain calm, even in a tense or hectic situation, and concentrate on the patient.

Therapeutic touch has been called a healing meditation because during the healing act the healer's brain wave pattern resembles those found in adept meditators. In some way this 'healing meditation' of the healer is transmitted to the patient who becomes relaxed as if they themselves were meditating.

Assessment

Although termed assessment, the second phase of therapeutic touch is not related in any way to traditional nursing or medical assessment or diagnosis. The healer simply passes his/her hands over the patient's body, not touching the skin surface but in the area immediately surrounding the person in what Krieger terms the 'human field' of the individual (p. 43).[13] The healer may experience changes in temperature in this field, 'heat and cold' and/or 'tingling', pressure, electric shocks or pulses. These sensations are thought to indicate changes or differences in the patient's energy flow which results from a state of imbalance and disease. Krieger describes the process as 'listening' to the patient with the palms of one's hands. These 'differences' in the patient's field may, according to Krieger, be due to a build-up of positive ions because 'Positive ion loading has been noted in crowded and congested locations where feelings of lethargy, headache, irritability etc have been noted to prevail' (p. 53).[13] The healer experiencing these areas of 'congestion' in the patient's field can relieve it by 'unruffling the field'.

Mobilising the energy field

This is the third phase of therapeutic touch healing, and is done by stroking or sweeping gestures of the healer's hands along the patient's body until the 'ruffle effect' or congestion is relieved, usually in a matter of minutes. The major purpose of this 'stroking phase' is to 'free' the bound energy — in other words, to get it moving and so facilitate the healing. It is common practice at the end of this phase of therapeutic touch for the healer to shake his/her hands or rinse them in water before proceeding to the concluding phase of directing energy to the patient. This shakes off any 'charges' picked up from the patient's energy field.

Directing energy

Directing energy to rebalance the energy field of the ill person can be achieved from the healer's own source of energy, or by moving energy from one place to another within the body and field force of the patient. Either way the healer should avoid being drained by the experience. The healer should see himself/herself as an open channel for flowing energy rather than a finite energy source. The aim of this phase is, according to Krieger 'to try to make both sides of the ill person's field 'feel the same' (p. 57).[13] Energy is therefore directed to the areas which felt 'different' during the assessment. If for example, the patient's knee felt 'hot' the healer places one hand above the knee and one below and mentally pictures the energy flowing to the affected joint. Some healers attempt to moderate the energy by imagining the energy to have, for example, a cooling quality. The healer may use a colour image to facilitate this — for example, blue is a sedating colour, red is an invigorating or stimulating one, and yellow is energising. Dolores Krieger, describing this process, writes 'I find that the easiest way for me to conceptualize a modulation of energy is in terms of colour. There are several reasons for this, but the most basic is that the colours we perceive are actually different wavelengths of energy' (p. 60).[13] The values ascribed to the colours appears to be pretty universal especially in relation to blue, red and yellow.

The healer thus directs the energy for, or to, the patient either by placing the hands on either side of the patient's body or by holding both hands above the patient until she feels that it is time to stop — usually about 15 minutes. She recognises that the time to stop is 'when there are not longer any cues: that is, relative to the body's symmetry there are now no perceivable differences bilaterally, between one side of the field and the other as one scans the healee's field' (p. 69).[13]

Observing the results

Although I have described the act of healing as outlined by Krieger and the concept of energy transfer that it involves, it has to be admitted, as she herself says, that quite frankly there is little in terms of quantifiable scientific evidence that this actually occurs. The mechanisms by which the laying on of hands produces beneficial results is at best poorly understood. But whatever one believes the source of healing to be, it is clear that the results of healing can be observed, and the mechanism by which it is achieved is open to exploration.

This exploration has to some extent been undertaken by American nurses who were students of Krieger at New York University. These nurses began to use therapeutic touch in their clinical practice and found that their patients said they felt more relaxed, calmer and more peaceful following the intervention. One PhD study by Patricia Heidt[15] provides research data to substantiate these subjective statements. Heidt's 90 volunteers were patients in a hospital cardiovascular unit of a large medical centre in New York. The patients were divided into three matched groups, each subject received an individual 5 minute period of intervention. The dependent variable of patient's anxiety was measured before and after the intervention.

One group received therapeutic touch using the four phases described above. The second group received casual touch through the taking of routine pulse rates at the patients' wrists, ankles and chest. The third group were not touched but were given 5 minutes focused conversation starting with 'Can you tell me how you are feeling today?' The patients in the therapeutic touch group experienced a highly significant reduction in state anxiety according to pre-test and post-test comparisons. And this was a markedly greater reduction in post-test anxiety scores than subjects who received intervention by casual touch or no touch at all.

It could be argued that this reduction in patients' anxiety and the sense of relaxation that accompanied it is a result of the nurses' hand movements. These movements or 'passes' could be hypnotic in themselves and so produce this effect, so another nurse researcher[16] tested this hypothesis. She compared the effect of real therapeutic touch with mimic therapeutic touch, that is, an intervention that mimics the movements of the nurse doing therapeutic touch but during which there is no attempt to centre, no intention to assess the subject, no attuning to the condition or the subject, and no direction of energy. Quinn videoed the nurses in both the 'real' and 'mimic' groups, and outside observers were unable to distinguish between them — in other words, they looked as though they were doing the same thing, but the results demonstrated that they were not. Based on the results of a self-administered pre-test and post-test questionnaire, Quinn was able to show a greater decrease in post-test state anxiety scores in subjects treated with 'real' therapeutic touch than in those treated with 'mimic' therapeutic touch.

The results of Quinn's study supports Krieger's assertion that therapeutic touch is a healing meditation in which the intention of the healer and the ability to remain 'centred' is a vital and necessary part of the therapy.

NURSING APPLICATION OF HEALING: THERAPEUTIC TOUCH

Therapeutic touch as taught by Krieger has been used in a wide variety of settings. One prison nurse, Joey Upland, has pioneered its use with jail inmates, working to heal their psychospiritual wounds alongside their physical needs, and this is a vital nursing act.

> Because any kind of loving touch that may soothe needs and prevent an inmate from further losing touch with basic human-ness is suspect and absent in this environment, the nurse becomes the provider of basic human nurture for the inmate, whether in the form of dispensing pills or a healing touch . . . Being centred and grounded in the prison environment a healer presents a powerful healing force.[17]

Upland describes the success she had in treating inmates with therapeutic touch and a number of similar examples of the beneficial use of therapeutic touch are also provided. One nurse described the use of therapeutic touch in the operating room where 'most people sense this type of non-physical stroking as being very soothing and conducive to relaxation. This physiological relaxation greatly benefits the induction of general anaesthesia'.[17]

Therapeutic touch may also be beneficial for the dying patient as adjunctive pain relief and emotional support. Mueller Jackson illustrates this aspect of her work with a 54-year-old leukaemia patient, Marilyn, suffering from unrelieved pain, depression and a feeling that she could not breathe.

> I asked her if I could put my hand on the place where it hurts and use a touch technique that some times works with pain such as hers. She agreed and I gently placed one hand on her back. I took her pulse with the other hand and timed her respirations. Pulse 96 and respirations were 58 per minute. I then began therapeutic touch. The assessment revealed to me an area of strong heat in the area of her pelvis and lower back and a tingling sensation radiating around her head. After several minutes she said the pain was 'letting up a bit', and that she felt a wave of heat 'kind of like sunlight' from head to toe. Her respirations had decreased to 28 per minute and her body was slowly uncurling from the tight position. After ten minutes her pulse was 60 and her hands rested comfortably at her sides. She said she felt much better and 'lighter' (p. 75).[17]

Mueller Jackson concluded that for Marilyn a course of therapeutic touch was useful not only as an adjunct to pain medication but it also 'produced a physiological relaxation and a decrease in anxiety which facilitated her movement through the grief process and it helped her to finish her business' (p. 78).[17]

Children as well as adults can benefit from therapeutic touch — Diana Tinnerin (supervisor of a paediatric unit) provides three case studies where therapeutic touch was found to reduce the clinical symptoms of fever, intestinal inflammation and purpora, and assisted with bone healing (p. 64).[17] In the case of Jamie who had grossly inflamed intestines from Henoch–Schönlein's purpura, she found that following a couple of therapeutic touch sessions Jamie had a virtually healed bowel: 'Clinically Jamie presented a bewildering picture. The physicians were mystified and could not explain the negative findings particularly when three days earlier his intestinal picture had been so glaringly poor.'

Finnerin continued to give therapeutic touch and 'within two days Jamie's symptoms began to subside and gradually they disappeared. The entire staff was astounded by the disappearance of symptoms and it was agreed that some unexplained factor was at work and needed further investigation' (p. 68).[17] Although much of the evidence for the effectiveness of healing on patients is anecdotal rather than 'scientific' evidence — it seems beyond reasonable doubt that healing provides an aid to relaxation and facilitates the patient's own recuperative powers.

THE EFFECTS OF HEALING ON THE CAREGIVER

The effects of stress in nursing are well recognised, from apathy to total 'burnout'. Increasingly this is so when nurses are expected to provide for the holistic needs of patients and carers without appropriate resources or a facilitating management structure and often with little encouragement to meet their own needs for 'nurturance and replenishment'.[18] The practice of healing provides one means of nurses meeting their own needs by 'focusing on the positive dimensions of their caregiver role'.[18]

In one study by Randolph (cited in Sandroff[19]) on the effects of therapeutic touch on the practitioners themselves, the latter found that their own health improved after they started to use therapeutic touch on their patients: 'She noticed that they managed to avoid some of the occupational hazards of nursing — exhaustion, depression, apathy and working on automatic' (p. 30).[19]

This positive outcome for the nurse healers may be due to their meditational practice during healing, to their expanded philosophy or to the feeling of close and effective communication with patients — but whatever the cause healing is clearly a positive two-way process.

The practice of healing appears to facilitate not only the patient's adjustment to stress but also the practitioner's state of health and view of the world. As one nurse puts it: 'I know for certain that using therapeutic touch has changed and continues to change me. Including alternative modalities of healing in one's practice requires a certain philosophy, and this change or expansion of philosophy pervades one's total existence' (p. 62).[17]

CONCLUSIONS

Healing is non-invasive, with only minimal possible side-effects (for example, feeling faint, or hypotensive), and uses one of the most fundamental communication skills of the nurse. It is therefore an eminently suitable therapy for nurses to incorporate into their care, with positive spinoffs for the nurse. In a time of accelerating medical costs, high technology and the recognition of medical sciences inability to 'cure all ills', as witness the AIDS epidemic — healing offers a way of emphasising the patient's unique human needs, and is a practical demonstration of the nurse's desire to care for and heal the individual, while recognising the interrelatedness of mind, body and spirit.

REFERENCES

1. Oojendijk, W.T.H., Mackenbach, J.P. and Limberger, H.H.B. What is better? An investigation into the use of, and satisfaction with complementary and official medicine in the Netherlands. The Netherlands Institute of Preventive Medicine and Technical Industrial Organisation (The Threshold Foundation, London, 1980).

2. Fulder, S.J. and Monro, R. The Status of Complementary Medicine in the United Kingdom (The Threshold Foundation, London, 1981).

3. Sherman, J. 'News Focus: Alternative Medicine: The Laying on of Hands'. Nursing Times (20 November 1985), pp. 18–19.

4. Harvey, D. The Power to Heal: An Investigation of Healing and the Healing Experience (The Aquarian Press, London, 1983).

5. MacManaway, B. and Turcan, J. *Healing* (Thorsons, Wellingborough, 1983).

6. Taylor-Reilly, D. 'Young Doctors' Views on Alternative Medicine', *British Medical Journal* (1983), 287, pp. 337–9.

7. British Medical Association 'Alternative Therapy: Report of the Board of Science and Education', *British Medical Association* (May 1986).

8. MacNutt, F. *Healing*, 5th edition (Bantam Books, London, 1979).

9. Pearce, I. *The Gate of Healing* (Neville Spearman, Jersey, 1983).

10. Krieger, D. 'Therapeutic Touch: The Imprimatur of Nursing', *American Journal of Nursing* (May 1975), pp. 784–7.

11. Krieger, D. *The Renaissance Nurse* (J.B. Lippincott Co., Philadelphia, 1981).

12. Krieger, D. 'Therapeutic Touch', *Mediscope: Manchester Medical Gazette* (1982), 61 (1), pp. 10–12. Manchester University.

13. Krieger, D. *The Therapeutic Touch: How to Use Your Hands to Help or to Heal* (Prentice Hall, Englewood Cliffs, New Jersey, 1979).

14. Bond, M. *Stress and Self Awareness* (Heinemann, London, 1986).

15. Heidt, P. 'Effect of Therapeutic Touch on Anxiety Level of Hospitalised Patients', *Nursing Research* (1981), 30 (1), pp. 32–7.

16. Quinn, J. 'Therapeutic Touch as Energy Exchange', *Advances in Nursing Science* (January 1984), pp. 42–9.

17. Borelli, M.D. and Heidt, P. *Therapeutic Touch* (Springer Publishing Co, New York).

18. Munley, A. 'Sources of Hospice Staff Stress and How to Cope with It', *Nursing Clinics of North America* (1985), 20 (2), pp. 343, 353.

19. Sandroff, R. 'The Sceptic's Guide to Therapeutic Touch', *Registered Nurse* (January 1980) pp. 26–9.

USEFUL ADDRESSES

Westbank Healing and Teaching Centres
Strathmiglo
Fife
Scotland
KY14 7QP
Telephone: 03376 233

British Alliance of Healing Associations
17 Fernwood
Hadleigh
Benfleet
Essex
SS7 2LT
Telephone: 0702 558430

College of Healing
Running Park
Croft Bank
West Malvern
Worcestershire
WR14 4BP
Telephone: 06845 3868

11

Biofeedback and Self-regulation

Chandra Patel

INTRODUCTION: WHAT IS BIOFEEDBACK?

When I first started using biofeedback in my research in 1973, it was hailed as a miraculous treatment for a wide variety of conditions like headaches, insomnia, cardiac arrythmias, hypertension, stroke, epilepsy, dysmenorrhagia, anxiety, backache, tinnitus, irritable bowel syndrome, asthma, reading disability; it was even reported to be a potential contraceptive method. It was considered a scientific breakthrough and was a subject of articles in *Science, Wall Street Journal, Playboy* and many newspapers. A paperback published in the United States in 1973[1] asserted that biofeedback is:

(1) an extraordinary technique which allows you control of the state of your health, happiness and wellbeing solely through the power of your mind;
(2) a spectacular scientific theory which has become fact in hospitals and laboratories across the country;
(3) a revolutionary method of getting quickly in touch with the inner self;
(4) a visionary technology which places the power for change and control in the hands of the individual and allows him to control his own destiny.

It is not the first time that we have heard of a panacea in medicine. Purging and bloodletting too had their era. We, in Britain, have learnt to be cautious through history, although at times this attitude of apathy and indifference has been equally damaging. Now that dust has settled, the therapy is considered neither sensational nor utopian. However, if used properly, it still represents a major breakthrough in the understanding and harnessing of our own healing or recuperative powers. It represents a control mechanism in which patients, through changes in their own behaviour and thoughts by an act of will, can learn to correct maladaptation in their own physiology.

Within health care, biofeedback offers nurses and many health care workers an opportunity to promote self-monitoring and self-training procedures in order to regulate and reduce a number of disorders, for example, essential hypertension, migraine, tension headaches and even cancers; these are discussed more fully below.

As both a treatment and preventive measure, nurses are perhaps ideally placed to play an important role in the health care team towards screening patients for preventable diseases and monitoring the progress of non-drug measures including biofeedback. Furthermore, by training in this procedure, daily nursing care could be extended to include the therapy and to encourage patients to become more self-reliant in the maintenance of their own health.

Biofeedback uses electronic instruments which, when connected to an individual, can measure, amplify and display one of several physiological processes on a moment-to-moment basis. Thus, internal informations not normally available to our usual five senses are literally fed back to the person connected in easily perceived and understood signals. These signals can take auditory forms like clicks and tones, or visual forms like digital readouts, analogue signal, lights or graphs and thus be directed to the command of the will.

For example, a patient with a tension headache is able to see or hear the level of tension in the back or front of his head through electromyographic feedback even before the head starts hurting, and by learning to reduce that tension he can learn to prevent headaches. Since reduced tension is also instantly displayed, the person can learn by trial and error appropriate thoughts and behaviour associated with reduced levels of muscle tension. Through other instruments people can learn to control brainwave patterns, blood pressure, sweat gland activity, skin temperature, heartbeats and so on.

Feedback mechanism is not new. It has been used in engineering for years, while feedback loops in the regulation of our physiological and endocrinological functions are well known. The oldest biofeedback instrument which was already known to us is a weighing machine. We are not able to perceive accurately the loss or gain of a few pounds in body weight, but with the scale we can monitor the effect of a diet and the knowledge of success reinforces our new

165

dietary habits. Voluntary control of physiological functions through yoga, meditation and breathing techniques are also well known. So why did it take so many years to develop biofeedback further to include voluntary control of autonomic functions in medicine?

HISTORY OF BIOFEEDBACK

The Russian physiologist, Pavlov, in his classical conditioning experiments on dogs had already shown that dogs can be made to salivate on the presentation of a gong if the gong had been repeatedly presented to them previously in association with food. An American psychologist, Skinner, had already demonstrated through operant conditioning techniques that animals can be made to learn new behaviours if such learning was properly rewarded, and we all knew that circus animals learn many external behaviours mediated by the skeletal muscles when rewarded with food. In the 1960s, Neal Miller, a psychologist from Rockefeller University in New York, and his colleagues, stunned the world when they successfully combined the above observations and used operant conditioning techniques in animals to control autonomic functions.

In the early experiment Miller and his colleagues showed that a water-deprived dog could be made to increase or decrease salivation if rewarded by water.[2] In order to see if autonomic functions could be controlled without the mediation of skeletal muscles in later experiments,[3] they curarised rats and rewarded the appropriate learning by electrical stimulation of the pleasure centre of the brain. Believe it or not, the rats very quickly learned to control functions that were rewarded. They could increase or decrease blood pressure, gastric secretion, urine formation, intestinal contraction, heart rate and carry out even more exotic tricks like blushing (vasodilatation) in one ear, but not in the other at the same time!

Further studies showed that even the magnitude of changes could be influenced by a 'shaping' procedure in which animals had to meet progressively more difficult criteria to obtain this reward.[4] Some of the rats involved in slowing the heart rate experiments with this 'shaping' procedure reduced their heart rates so much that cardiac arrest occurred! Reduction in blood pressure by 30 mmHg was quite common. This led to the opening of the Pandora's box and eventually the feeling that if rats can do it so can humans. Neal Miller said: 'I believe in this respect they are as smart as rats.'

DEVELOPMENT OF ELECTRONIC INSTRUMENTS AND THEIR RELEVANCE TO PSYCHOSOMATIC ILLNESS

An infant learns to smile or walk through trial and error. The mother reinforces correct behaviour by hugging or feeding. A child learns to play the piano because he can see the keys and hear the tune, and through trial and error he learns to press the right keys to get the right tune while the teacher's praise or obtaining examination grades reinforces the learning.

But how can we learn to control our blood pressure or change our heart rates if we cannot see or hear them? The answer was not too difficult for our highly developed technology. Electronic instruments were developed so that we can actually see or hear our blood pressure, heart rate, brainwave pattern, muscle tension, sweat gland activity, skin temperature and so on. Since changes in these activities are at the roots of anxiety, tension and psychosomatic ills, it became apparent that it would be wise to listen to these signals and learn to control them rather than taking tranquillisers, sleeping pills or painkillers.

AETIOLOGY OF PSYCHOSOMATIC ILLNESS

Whenever we are confronted with a novel or stressful situation, our mind and body responds by arousal or alertness to take action. The subconscious also searches through the brain's memory files and compares data and association previously stored. Is the situation new? Is it something to worry about? Is it dangerous? Can I cope with it? What actions are necessary? And within a matter of milliseconds decisions are reached. If the situation is coded to be pleasant, or adequate coping abilities are recognised in one's repertoire, the body systems are not further alerted and the state of initial arousal subsides. If on the other hand it is thought to be unpleasant or threatening in some way, or effective coping responses are not identified, the body systems of nerves and muscles are further alerted into readiness for defence, breathing becomes erratic, muscles become tense, the skin perspires, the heart speeds up, the skin vessels become constricted, blood pressure rises, and blood is diverted to the muscles and brain which becomes extremely alert ready to make swift decisions.

Most circumstances however are not life-or-death situations, but dramatic and rapidly moving patterns of mental emotional demands

167

of social, economic, occupational or political pressures which can be solved without the expensive body–mind response or undue apprehension or anxiety. However, the subconscious registers these problems as dangers and physiological response is mobilised. When cumulations occur over months or years, anxiety and tension are brought into awareness and one of many psychosomatic illnesses may appear. By this time, however, we have become unsure of their sources, and are unable to attribute them to any single source of fear or anxiety. This is one of the reasons why it is difficult to establish the link between stress and psychosomatic symptoms. Unfortunately, the need to establish the cause before rational logical treatment can be offered has led to unnecessary suffering. The strange fact is that even though orthodox medicine will not accept stress as the basis of psychosomatic illnesses, it happily accepts the use of tranquillisers without any question.

If we can uncover abnormal responses of the mind and body through biofeedback instruments long before the disease becomes established or disabling, there is a hope that we may be able to prevent the long-term effect of the emotions on the body in a most efficient and inexpensive way. These are the premises on which biofeedback treatment is based.

TYPES OF BIOFEEDBACK INSTRUMENTS

Galvanic skin resistance or GSR

Skin has an amazing ability to communicate the state of the mind. It is used by police and personnel departments in a lie detection test during which the electrical capacities of the skin communicate information about our personal thoughts, feelings, fear and anxiety and give us away. No matter what the person *says*, the skin does not lie. Skin resistance biofeedback is different from any other form of feedback. In heart rate, blood pressure, muscle tension, brainwave pattern feedback, the respective machines give information strictly limited to those organs or functions while skin primarily talks about the complexity of the mind and not about the skin itself. This vast potential can be exploited to solve emotional problems and control hidden responses of the mind despite the fact that its language is not always clearly understood.

The instrument consists of a box and a length of wire leading to two surface electrodes which can be secured, for example, to two fingers. By applying a small amount of electric current, it is possible to measure the resistance offered by the skin to the passage of the current and see how the skin's electrical activity surges in intensity with emotion and excitement and falls with quiescence and relaxation. The electrical behaviour of the skin reflects the changes that occur during the resumption of sweat and changes in the permeability of the cell membrane to various ions of the mineral elements in the skin. The electrical activity mirrors the mind's response to emotions — anxiety, fear, anger, passion or delight and thus allows us to listen to the deep within and expand limits of our self-knowledge. Its signals can be converted into a graph, recorded on moving paper or, more commonly, in the tones or clicks of differing pitch, loudness and intervals. The more realistic information is thus brought out of the subconscious into the realm of consciousness to be confronted and used for diagnostic purpose or subjected to volitional control. The result is mind controlling the mind, thoughts controlling the thoughts. This instrument can be used for practically any psychosomatic condition.

Electromyography (EMG) or muscle tension biofeedback

When adults resort to alcohol or youngsters resort to other heavy drugs, they are acknowledging unacceptable or uncomfortable degrees of tension and the need to get 'loosened up'. When a patient complaints to the nurse or physician that she is so uptight she is unable to sleep, she is describing tension in the muscles; and when the doctor or well wishers tell one to relax, they are saying that tension is at the root of one's disease or symptoms. Yet most people will deny that they are tense. If they are asked to rate tension from 1 to 10 with 1 being most relaxed and 10 being extremely tense, most will rate themselves with a tension score of 2 and 3, or 4 at the most.

The problem is one of adaptation. The body responds to anxiety or nervousness by bracing some muscles. Stiff muscles send signals to the brain and one becomes aware of the tension. However, this feeling is only temporary as the brain fails to take notice of this feeling if the state of tension continues for any length of time, and we soon forget that we are tense. A more convincing analogy is with adaptation to a sense of smell. If we enter a room with a strong odour, we immediately notice it. But if we stay in the room for any length of time, the odour becomes less and less apparent because the brain accommodates. Without outside indicators of how uptight the muscles are, learning to relax can become a long, slow, unrewarding process.

Even though muscle tension is not an automatic function, biofeedback of the muscles activity allows us to look at the real level of muscle tension, and gives us the opportunity to reduce tension by learning to relax. The relaxation training is thus made more accurate, and learning not only becomes more fun but also a refreshingly challenging task.

The subject is asked to sit or recline in a comfortable chair and small discs like electrodes are pasted on the surface of chosen muscles (for example, frontalis muscles in the case of tension headaches). The electrical activity of the muscle is picked up, amplified and conveyed back as some form of visual or auditory signal. In the latter, which is a more common form, a tone tells you how tense or relaxed the muscle is. The higher the tone, the greater the tension — and then it is the patient's job to lower the pitch of the tone by relaxing. Sometimes muscle activity over a short period of time is added and displayed as a number and the task is to try to reduce the number displayed to lower and lower figures. Thus the machine instantly tells both the patient and the therapist not only the level of activity, but also the rate at which it is changing. In the beginning, the therapist makes the task easier so that the patient is able to recognise even small reductions in the level of tension. But as he becomes more expert, the therapist makes it more and more difficult for him to lower the tone.

The process can also be reversed in which the subject tries to increase the tone by increasing the electrical activity of the muscle under the sensing electrode, or made even more complex in which he can inhibit activity of most muscle fibres except a single motor representing one motor neurone in the spinal cord and its nerve fibrils carrying information to and from the muscle cells they supply.

John Basmajian, a neuroanatomist from Canada, has been a pioneer in this field. In 1969 he declared that human beings can quickly, in a matter of 15–20 minutes, isolate only one motor unit from the population of perhaps 100 or 200 within an area of a tiny electrode, and fire it at will suppressing all other units; they can then suppress the one they started with, pick up another one, train to fire that and then suppress it — all by the command of the will.[5]

Theoretically such instruments can be used to treat many

conditions in which muscle tension level is high, ranging from tension headache or local muscle spasms to cerebral palsy. People, who clench their teeth during sleep so much that they wear out their teeth (bruxism) can be helped if they sleep with electrodes stuck over their jaw muscles. When the muscles contract during sleep, the machine on registering the tension will give out an auditory signal and wake the patient up. Of course the patient needs to learn relaxation as well. Machines can be used in learning more complicated tasks like relaxing one set of muscle fibres while tensing the other, when muscle coordination is deranged in conditions like stammering, wry neck or faecal incontinence. Learning to activate muscle fibres has been used in neuromuscular rehabilitation in strokes.

Electroencephalographic (EEG) biofeedback

There is nothing more intriguing and awe-inspiring about the human body than the intricate workings of the human brain. Some 20 billion brain cells are packed into the skull surpassing the capacity of any telephone exchange or even the most complicated computer system. The revelations of its electrical energy, called brainwaves or electro-encephalogram (EEG), by biofeedback and human ability to control the pattern at will is the most startling of the discoveries. This electric energy not only moves the pen back and forth on the recording paper but can even be used to drive electronic devices, to bring on light or sound signals.

Different states of mind, thoughts and perspectives are associated with different wave forms: alert brain, for example, is associated with beta-waves which are flat and occur relatively fast at the rate of 13–28 cycles per second. Alpha-waves are high amplitude waves occurring at 8–12 cycles/s when the person is relaxed with his/her eyes closed or is in the so-called twilight zone before falling asleep. During meditation, alpha-waves appear in abundance. Theta-waves are slow waves occurring at the rate of 4–7 cycles/s, are larger than alpha-waves and occur during drowsiness, dreaming, and during assimilation of new information. Children and geniuses sometimes show theta-waves during their waking state and this seems to represent creative states. Very slow delta-waves at 1–3 cycles/s occur during sleep. It must be remembered that this classification is an oversimplification of the subject, and hundreds of variations of each wave form, combination and permutation are quite common.

171

Joe Kamiya[6] introduced alpha EEG biofeedback in which production of every alpha-wave produced a click. The function of the subject learning to produce alpha-waves was to bring on as many clicks as possible. Kamiya reported that those subjects with prior experience of meditation were the best learners. Later it was found that successful learning of alpha-waves was accompanied by increased susceptibility to hypnosis. People capable of vivid visual imagery were also found to have large quantities of alpha-waves. Since people with special behaviour problems and users of drugs like marijuana and heroin have predominant wave patterns slightly slower than alpha-waves, use of alpha feedback is contraindicated in these people.

As production of large numbers of alpha-waves was described to be associated with feelings of pleasantness, tranquillity or relaxation, its application has been in the relief of anxiety or in the facilitation of relaxation. The most popular attraction, however, in alpha feedback is to facilitate learning of meditation since practitioners of yoga or Zen meditation are reported to have a 'high alpha state'. It has even been suggested that EEG biofeedback can be used to bring at least some psychic ability under voluntary control. Another promising area is prevention or control of epilepsy. Learning to produce a narrow band of 12–14 cycles/s over sensory motor cortex was successfully used to reduce epileptic seizures[7] and hyperkinesia in hyperactive children.[8] Further studies to confirm these findings are necessary.

Thermal feedback

It was suggested that some of the yogis who live in the cold climates of the Himalayas learn to voluntarily control their body temperature, and in one scientific study a yogi was reported to have produced visible perspiration over his forehead within a matter of 1½ minutes of turning his mind inwardly. When skin temperature biofeedback machines were developed and the curtain of mysticism was removed, it became apparant that people with little or no prior experience of thermal feedback could learn to significantly raise the temperature of their hands within a matter of days. If meditation or relaxation is combined with temperature feedback, people are likely to learn temperature control faster than when given feedback alone where they are left to devise their own strategies to raise skin temperature. The most common temperature feedback is combined with autogenic training[9] in which people use self-suggestion phrases like 'my arms and legs are warm'.

Thermal biofeedback combined with autogenic training have been reported to be beneficial in migraine,[10] Raynaud's disease,[11] and general anxiety state, or in improving patient's belief in their own capacity to control physiological functions before efforts are made to control specific conditions. This procedure could also have possible application for the nursing care of the elderly, or patients likely to be physically susceptible to temperature fluctuations, as in hypertension, for example.

Feedback of rate and rhythm of the heart

We are not normally aware of the constant rhythmic activity of the heart except during rare, quiet occasions when the chest wall is resting against a bed or pillow. Such awareness of our heart beat or palpitations can be distressing and we may even change our position to make the heart beats go away from our consciousness. Exercise and strong emotions are other occasions when we may become conscious of our heart beats. Long before science had discovered the connection between emotions and the heart's rhythmic activity, poets and writers had already endowed the heart with an ability to express every human emotion — sadness, fear, despair, oppression, sickness, understanding, passion or jealousy. Feelings of loss during bereavement leading to death from a broken heart have already been shown in scientific studies.

The heart is supplied by two sets of nerves: sympathetic and parasympathetic, each with the ability to oppose the function of the other and thus helping to maintain the balance in the life-support system. Sympathetic overactivity or parasympathetic inhibition during stressful situations can lead the heart to beat rapidly or erratically.[12] A diseased heart is particularly sensitive to neuro-hormonal changes, and minor rhythm disturbance may herald a more serious variety of arrhythmia and even death.[13] Feedback of the heart's rate or rhythm thus allows the individual to exert personal control, and studies have reported reduction in both the frequency of premature ventricular contractions (PVCs), and in ventricular rate in atrial fibrillation, and in ventricular parasystolic rhythm;[14-17] when biofeedback training was combined with relaxation training, reduction in PVCs during sleep was maintained.[18] Clinical significance of these observations has not yet been established.

Blood pressure biofeedback

Elevated blood pressure is so common that it may affect as much as 40 per cent of the adult population in developed countries. In 90–95 per cent of the cases, no cause is known and they are assigned to the category of essential hypertension. Its relentless progress leads to a variety of complications frequently encountered in daily nursing care, and includes strokes, coronary heart attacks, congestive heart failure, renal failure and peripheral vessel disease. In severe hypertension, drug treatment is known to reduce most complications except coronary heart disease. As a result, efforts are being made to identify those with mild hypertension with a view to controlling blood pressure before the development of atherosclerosis which underlines most of the complications. In a mild hypertension trial involving some 1800 patients,[19] drug treatment unfortunately did not reduce deaths or coronary heart disease. Antihypertensive drugs also led to uncomfortable side-effects like impotence, gout, diabetes, cold fingers, depression and nightmares.[20] If mild hypertension can be controlled without drugs, it may offer many advantages.

In general, drug treatment does not take into account that increased tension in the artery also reflects increased psychological and social tension in patients' lives. This process is so insidious that by the time hypertension is detected, the patient is not aware of any specific tension, and even if he tries to recollect and describe them the physician very quickly dismisses them saying that there is no evidence of stress playing any role in the aetiology of hypertension. It was not until the revelation of failures of drugs to prevent complications that the medical profession began to pay some attention to alternative medicine.

Shapiro and his colleagues from Harvard Medical School developed a blood pressure biofeedback instrument consisting of an arm cuff with an embedded crystal microphone placed over the brachial artery. The cuff is inflated to a median systolic pressure so that Korotoff sounds are picked up only 50 per cent of the time. Each time blood pressure is either increased or decreased by a predetermined criterion, a feedback signal was produced in the form of a light to indicate in which direction the response of the blood pressure was changing. Medical students who volunteered for this early experiment were asked to bring on lights, each of which signified a correct response. After 20 correct responses the student was rewarded by presentation of a slide (for example depicting a nude female for male students!) or money. The students on average were able to increase blood pressure by 0.6 mmHg or decrease it to about 4 mmHg.[21] Although these changes were statistically significant, their clinical meaningfulness was in doubt and it was quite apparent that the changes produced by rats were not matched by human subjects. Subsequent interviews of the best learners also failed to identify any consistent cognitive or behavioural strategies.[22]

It became clear that biofeedback instruments merely produce the information about certain physiological functions and were useful in allowing the subjects to respond more accurately. But the development of a behaviour that can produce therapeutic changes in physiology is more important than the biofeedback instruments, since the instruments are to be abandoned once the training is over, while the behaviour has to become a part of life if the therapeutic gain is to become permanent. To quote Skinner,[23] 'What is needed is a technology of behaviour. The human problems cannot be solved by physical and biological technology alone.'

THE ROLE OF MEDITATION AND MEDITATION-BASED TECHNIQUES

The desire to control one's physiology is not a new concept conjured up by the biofeedback scientist for the first time. To be able to control one's own destiny, behaviour, states of consciousness and physiology has been a pervasive feature of human nature. It has taken many religious, cultic and non-cultic forms. Various yoga techniques including breathing, deep muscle relaxation, and meditation as a means to self-regulation are probably the most ancient.[24] Progressive muscle relaxation as popularised by Jacobson,[25] in which each group of muscles is tensed before relaxing has also been used. Autogenic training,[9] in which simple phrases are used autosuggestively to produce a deeply relaxed state, or specific formula to induce a specific physiological state, is also used extensively in conjunction with biofeedback instruments. In fact, biofeedback machines are hardly ever used alone nowadays.

Scientific evaluation

Biofeedback, with or without the addition of relaxation, meditation, autogenic training or stress management in which brief relaxation is practised during a stressful environment, has been extensively

175

evaluated in certain conditions. Those in which such 'non-dry' methods are showing promise are reviewed below.

Tension headache

It is generally assumed that there is no scientific evidence that increased tension in the muscles around the head is present in patients who have tension headaches.[26] Despite this, several experiments using EMG biofeedback showed significant benefits compared to medication,[27] attention placebo,[28] or self-relaxation.[29] Later studies, however, showed that biofeedback was not superior to proper relaxation training.[26,27,29] That some permanent changes in behaviour are necessary is suggested by the fact that benefits were maintained during follow-up in some studies[28,30,31] but not in others.[32] Learning to reappraise environmental situations, and hence one's reactions to them, was found to be superior to EMG biofeedback in one study.[33] The subjects in this study were, however, led to believe that the effects of therapy would be delayed for some time, thus the effect of *belief* was more powerful than the possible physiological changes.

In one study, EMG biofeedback was compared with diazepam.[34] During the trial period both were equally effective, but during the follow-up period, when neither diazepam nor biofeedback sessions were continued, headaches returned in the diazepam group, but the EMG biofeedback group was able to maintain the benefits. Thus it is clear that for long-term benefits, some form of behavioural changes are necessary, and biofeedback may act as an aid for learning these behavioural changes. Long-term medications have no place in the management of tension headaches.

Migraine

Many nurses, doctors and patients believe that stress and tension are implicated in migraine. The actual mechanism is not properly understood, but is thought to be vascular instability of extracranial vessels triggered by sympathetic overreactivity. Initial vasoconstriction leads to aura while later dilatation is responsible for the typical headaches. Two types of biofeedback instruments are generally used: the most common is temperature feedback from the hand to enable subjects to warm their hands — this was based on observations of some migraine patients that their hands felt cold prior to migraine attacks, and those who were learning to raise hand temperature in early voluntary-control experiments reported reductions in migraine;[35] the second type is aimed at controlling the size of the temporal artery since its dilatation is considered to underlie the painful aspect of a migraine headache.

Research studies in general suggest that temperature feedback does reduce intensity, duration and frequency of headaches. There is little reason to believe that it is an essential component of such treatment because relaxation training was slightly more effective than temperature feedback in one study,[36] while in another study feedback involving simultaneous cooling of the forehead, in addition to variety of other biofeedback techniques including EMG and EEG alpha feedback, were equally and modestly effective.[37] Other studies have produced conflicting results.

The use of temporary artery size feedback was also reported to reduce migraine in some studies;[38] but its superiority over temperature feedback has not been established.[39] Temperature feedback is usually combined with autogenic training in which the patient himself suggests that his limbs are becoming relaxed, and warm or extensive imageries are used such as imagining lying under hot sun or sitting in front of a fire. Several studies have shown that benefit persists during follow-up up to one year.[36,37,40] A combination of systematic desensitisation, assertiveness training and relaxation was more effective than relaxation alone in intractable migraine.[41] Although there has been no direct comparison of biofeedback or behavioural treatment with pharmacological therapy, most patients involved in the above studies represent treatment failures to drug therapy. It may be that a proportion of patients with infrequent migraine attacks can be satisfactorily controlled on drug treatment before or during attacks, but there still remains a sizeable number of patients who are not satisfactorily controlled. In these patients biofeedback or behavioural treatment can be suitable choices and may be preferred to long-term prophylactic medications.

Essential hypertension

It will never be possible to prove beyond reasonable doubt that stress is causally related to essential hypertension. However, there is sufficient circumstantial evidence which suggests that psychological factors are involved. Early promise of blood pressure control through blood pressure feedback[42-44] was not fulfilled in some of the later studies.[45-48] On the other hand, relaxation or hypertension combined with some form of biofeedback were found to be more effective than either procedure alone.[49-52]

Patel and her colleagues have shown that a combination of relaxation, meditation, breathing, exercise, GSR biofeedback and stress management lead to clinically meaningful reduction in both medicated[53-55] and unmedicated[56] hypertensive patients. Such behavioural treatment not only enables patients to take reduced or no medication, but may also lower the chances of cardiovascular complications.[57] Similar reductions in blood pressure have been reported in studies using relaxation only.[58-60] Irvine[62] found the relaxation and stress management package developed by Patel more effective, compared with elaborate control procedure of mobility exercises which matched in complexity number of attendance, expectations and home practice.

Anxiety states

EMG biofeedback, usually combined with relaxation or autogenic training, has been extensively used in generalised anxiety state in systematic desensitisation procedures for specific phobias, initially as a guide to rapidly learning successful relaxation, and then as an acute monitor of tension during visualisation of scenes from the 'fear hierarchy'.[63-65] Patients are often surpised to see how high are their levels of tension while they thought they were satisfactorily relaxed. Similarly, biofeedback machines would register tension during exposure to 'fear hierarchy' while patients report that they are still relaxed.[63] EMG biofeedback has been found to be more effective than psychotherapy[66] or cognitive monitoring[67] in reducing anxiety. In one study, EMG biofeedback was found to be superior to diazepam (Valium).[68]

Cancer

This is a relatively new subject in which biofeedback is finding its most humane and yet exciting place. It is an issue laden with understandably emotional overtones, and it is unlikely that randomised controlled trials to evaluate the contribution of biofeedback in overcoming cancer is ever likely to be possible, but a number of case studies are revealing the phenomenal power of the mind.

It is believed that stress, involving particularly feelings of loss, helplessness and hopelessness in childhood or long before the clinical manifestations, is a precursor of cancerous growth. Even if there is disagreement as to whether or not stress causes cancer, there is general agreement that the body's ability to fight cancer is hindered by stress as the body's immune defences are compromised by it.

A typical treatment package involves learning to control various physiological responses like raising hand temperatures, reducing muscle tension or increasing alpha brainwaves, using a variety of biofeedback instruments combined with breathing, relaxation and meditation techniques. Biofeedback enables the patient to understand the hidden power of the mind to heal ourselves. Once the patient has made up his/her mind to fight cancer at all costs, he/she is further helped to decide upon a strategy in which he/she visualises, through imagination, the actual location of his/her cancer, and views the growth in the form of an evil (like a dragon, for example), and cancer cells as disorganised, weak, stupid and confused; at the same time he/she can visualise the immune defence system of white cells in the forms of strength like white knights or brave warriors in great numbers surging towards the cancer and destroying it, bit by bit, until it is completely demolished and disappears from the visual image. The process is repeated daily, or even twice a day, always starting with breathing exercises and relaxation.

It is important that the imagery is realistic and appealing to the individual if he/she is to believe in its power with utter faith and hope. This was borne out in a story told by one patient, a 9-year-old boy with an inoperable brain tumour which had partially paralysed the left side of his body.[69] He decided to fight the disease, but found a commercial tape of visualisation for cancer patients adult-orientated and thoroughly boring. So he and the therapist, Patricia Norris from the Menninger Foundation in the United States made a tape with convincing sound effects and dialogue in which the boy visualised himself as Blue Leader, the leader of a squadron of a fighter plane, his brain as a solar system, his cancer as invading planetoids entering his solar system and threatening its existence. He visualised simultaneously his white cells and other immune defences as lasers and torpedoes with which the squadron leader of the fighter plane was armed. The therapist's role was one of ground control, and by this device they maintained constant dialogue during visualisation of the battle scene.

The procedure is not easy by any means, as the battle is real, riddled with victories and setbacks, hits and misses. Maintaining self-confidence, courage, faith and hope are necessary and daily visualisation has to continue until the enemy is completely defeated and has disappeared from the visual scene. The boy fought daily for one year until he was unable to locate the tumour in his mind's eye; his muscle-power on the left side of his body was re-established, and brain scans carried out afterwards confirmed that the tumour was not detectable.

It is important to make a point that self-regulation therapy for any condition can be (and in cases of cancer must be) as advised by specialists, continued along with conventional treatment like radiation or chemotherapy. There is no conflict. In fact, if you combine mental imagery in which every bit of radiation or chemotherapy is directed to destroy cancer cells, it can potentiate their therapeutic effects and minimise their side-effects.

BIOFEEDBACK AND THE CHANGING ROLE OF THE NURSE

A recent report from the Royal College of Physician's Faculty of Community Physicians implied that we are one of the sickest nations of the developed world with a top place in the league table for heart diseases, chest diseases, cancers, preventable infections and accidents caused by drunk driving. They not only cause premature deaths, but also account for the majority of the total deaths and disability in the country. At the root of it all is the typical apathetic attitude of the people that their health is not within their personal control and that they must put their lives in the hands of medical experts when ill. Such attitudes have been fostered by the medical profession which wants to continue to relish the high and mighty position from the top of the pedestal where people put them in the first place.

Such a role may have been appropriate decades ago when the main causes of death and suffering were from diseases like smallpox, polio, diphtheria, cholera, typhoid, tuberculosis, pneumonia or meningitis. However, many of these diseases have either been eradicated or largely controlled by the dedicated work of pioneers who introduced hygienic measures like pure water, clean air, nutritious food, better housing, efficient sanitation, and developed immunisation procedures, antibiotics and chemotherapy. The patterns of illness have changed now, where stress and stress-related behaviours like smoking, drinking, overeating, and rebellion against authority are responsible for the majority of deaths and disability. Our health care delivery system must also change if we are to prevent premature deaths and promote the nation's health.

The belief that illness is something that befalls us as a result of our misfortune, and that the doctors will give pills or carry out surgery, and nurses will care for us until we are almost better is so deeply ingrained that there is a generalised reluctance on our part to take responsibility for looking after our own health. This was borne out very well in a large European Heart Disease Prevention Project in which some 60 000 men from the United Kingdom, Belgium, Poland and Italy took part.[70] Half of the men were given advice to stop smoking, to eat less fat in the diet to lose weight, to increase exercise, and to have high blood pressure (if present) treated by drugs. The other half were left alone. There was evidence of some reduction in all-cause mortality and incidence of coronary heart disease in Belgium. In Italy and Poland as many men in the intervention group lost weight, took up jogging, stopped smoking and changed their diets; but in the United Kingdom, the men continued the life and mortality pattern just as before. Nothing changed. The medical profession was surprised, but had to acknowledge the fact that the men in the United Kingdom failed to take the doctor's advice.

It is important that, as members of health care teams, we initiate new approaches to meet current health needs. People will have to take responsibility to look after their own health, but such responsibility cannot be delegated by mere words of advice. Nurses and health workers must evolve creative ways through which responsibility for health can be shifted to those whose health it is. Biofeedback and meditation seem to be an eminent means by which to produce an effective interface, as their main function is to instil a belief in people of their ability to confront events in their lives by convincingly demonstrating to them their power to change physiological functions by behavioural or cognitive means. The responsibility of getting people to participate in their health care is not the job of just one faction of the medical profession, but the business of every man and woman in health care.

The primary health care team is ideally placed for instigating preventive measures, but general practitioners cannot do this alone. Hospital and community nurses, general practice nurses, health visitors, and other members of the team must share in the responsibility shoulder to shoulder. The idea of a nurse practitioner or physician assistant (a nurse who trains further to carry out most of the routine jobs undertaken by the primary care physicians) did not take root in this country due to reluctance on both sides to change, but without creative changes we shall not be able to change disappointing statistics.

CONCLUSIONS

Biofeedback offers nurses the potential to play a more active role in screening for preventable diseases and help prevent them, take major burdens of caring for people with chronic conditions like hypertension, or participate in more humane care of people with psychosomatic diseases and even more serious conditions like cancer. In doing so, we would not only reduce deaths and disability, but also improve the physical, psychological and social wellbeing of the people we serve.

The recent, overwhelming and positive response to the Nursing Times Holistic Conferences in 1984 and 1986 indicate that nurses and many allied health care workers wish to develop their own knowledge of complementary therapies. In addition, they are aware of the potential health benefits many therapies could offer patients in terms of illness prevention and treatment.

The rapid and widespread interest shown by nurses may reflect as awareness that we must be more prepared to meet the demands of our patients — for more time, less prescriptions, more effective communication, and more say in the care of their own health.

REFERENCES

1. Karlins, M. and Andrews, L.M. *Biofeedback: Turning on the Power of Your Mind* (Warner Books, New York, 1972).

2. Miller, N.E. and Carmona, A. 'Modification of a Visceral Response: Salivation in Thirsty Dogs by Instrument Training with Water Reward'. *Journal of Comparative Physiology and Psychology* (1969), 63, pp. 1–6.

3. Miller, N.E. 'Learning of Visceral and Glandular Responses'. *Science* (1969), 163, pp. 434–45.

4. Miller, N.E. and Dicara, L.V. 'Instrumental Learning of Heart Rate Changes in Curarized Rats: Shaping and Specificity of Discriminative Stimulus'. *Journal of Comparative Physiology and Psychology* (1967), 63, pp. 12–19.

5. Basmajian, J.V. 'Control of Individual Motor Units'. *American Journal of Physical Medicine* (1967), 46, pp. 1247–14, 440.

6. Kamiya, J. 'Operant Control of the EEG Alpha Rhythm and Some of its Respected Effects of Consciousness', in C.T. Tarts (ed.) *Altered States of Consciousness* (Wiley, New York, 1969).

7. Sterman, M.B. and Friar, L. 'Suppression of Seizures in an Epileptic Following Sensorimotor EEG Feedback Training'. *Journal of Electroencephalography and Clinical Neurophysiology* (1972), 33, pp. 89–95.

8. Shouse, M.N. and Lubar, J.F. 'Operant Conditioning of EEG Rhythms and Ritalin in the Treatment of Hyperkinesis'. *Biofeedback and Self-regulation* (1979), 4, pp. 299–312.

9. Shultz, J.H. and Luthe, W. *Autogenic Therapy*, Vols. I–VI. (Grune and Stratton, New York, 1969).

10. Sargent, J.D., Walters, E.D. and Green, E.E. 'Psychosomatic Self-regulation of Migraine Headaches'. *Seminars in Psychiatry* (1973), 5, pp. 415–28.

11. Surwit, R.S. 'Behavioural Treatment of Raynaud's Disease', in R.S. Sunwit, R.B. Williams, A. Steptoe and R. Biergner (eds) *Behavioural Treatment of Disease* (Plenum Press, New York, 1982).

12. Teggart, P., Gibbons, D. and Sommerville, W. 'Some Effects of Motor Car Driving on the Normal and Abnormal Heart'. *British Medical Journal* (1969), 4, pp. 130–4.

13. Corbalan, R., Verrier, R. and Lown, B. 'Psychologic Stress and Ventricular Arrhythmias During Myocardial Infarction in Conscious Dogs'. *American Journal of Cardiology* (1974), 39, pp. 692–6.

14. Weiss, T. and Engel, B.T. 'Operant Conditioning of Heart Rate in Patients with Premature Ventricular Contractions'. *Psychosomatic Medicine* (1971), 33, pp. 301–21.

15. Bleeker, E.R. and Engel, B.T. 'Learned Control of Ventricular Rate in Patients with Atrial Fibrillation'. *Seminars in Psychiatry* (1973), 5, pp. 461–74.

16. Pickering, T. and Gorham, G. 'Learned Heart Rate Control by a Patient with Ventricular Parasystolic Rhythm'. *Lancet* (1975), 1, pp. 252–3.

17. Pickering, T.D. and Miller, N.E. 'Learned Voluntary Control of Heart Rate and Rhythm on Two Subjects with Premature Ventricular Contractions'. *British Heart Journal* (1977), 39, pp. 152–9.

18. Benson, H., Alexander, S. and Feldman, C.L. 'Decreased Premature Ventricular Contractions Through the Use of Relaxation Response in Patients with Ischaemic Heart Disease'. *Lancet* (1975), 2, pp. 380–2.

19. The Medical Research Council Working Party. 'MRC Trial of Treatment of Mild Hypertension. Principal Results'. *British Medical Journal* (1985), 291, pp. 97–104.

20. The Medical Research Council Working Party. 'Adverse Reaction to Bendrofluazide and Propranolol in the Treatment of Mild Hypertension'. *Lancet* (1981), 2, pp. 543–63.

21. Shapiro, D., Tursky, B. and Schwartz, G.E. 'Control of Blood Pressure in Man by Operant Conditioning'. *Circulation Research*, Suppl. 2, 26 and 27: 127–32.

22. Schwartz, G.E. and Shapiro, D. 'Biofeedback and Essential Hypertension: Current Findings and Theoretical Concerns'. *Seminars in Psychiatry* (1973), 5, pp. 493–502.

23. Skinner, B.F. *Beyond Freedom and Dignity* (Bantam, New York, 1971).

24. Patel, C. 'Yogic Therapy', in R.L. Woolfolk and P. Lehrer (eds) *The Principles and Practice of Stress Management* (Guildford Press, New York, 1984), pp. 70–107.

25. Jacobson, E. *Progressive Muscle Relaxation*, 2nd edn (University of Chicago Press, Chicago, 1938).

26. Martin, P.R. and Matthews, A.M. 'Tension Headache: Psychophysiological Investigation and Treatment'. *Journal of Psychosomatic Research* (1978), 22, pp. 389–99.

27. Cox, D.J., Freundlich, A. and Meyer, R.G. 'Differential Effectiveness of Electromyographic Feedback, Verbal Relaxation Instructions and Medication Placebo with Tension Headaches'. *Journal of Consultant and Clinical Psychology* (1975), 433, pp. 892–8.

28. Holroyd, D.A. and Andrasik, F. 'Coping and the Self-control of Chronic Tension Headache'. *Journal of Consultant and Clinical Psychology* (1980), 46, pp. 1036–45.

29. Haynes, S.N., Griffin, P., Mooney, D. and Parise, M. 'Electromyographic Biofeedback and Relaxation Instructions in the Treatment of Muscle Contraction Headaches'. *Behavioural Therapy* (1975), 6, pp. 672–8.

30. Budzynski, T.H., Stoyva, J.M., Adler, C.S. and Mullaney, E.J. 'EMG Biofeedback and Tension Headache: A Controlled Outcome Study'. *Psychosomatic Medicine* (1973), 35, pp. 484–96.

31. Hart, J.D. and Chichanski, K.A. 'A Comparison of Frontal EMG Biofeedback and Neck EMG Biofeedback in the Treatment of Muscle-contraction Headache'. *Biofeedback and Self-Regulation* (1981), 6, pp. 63–74.

32. Cram, J.R. 'EMG Biofeedback Training and the Treatment of Tension Headaches: A Systematic Analysis of Treatment Components'. *Behavioural Therapy* (1980), 11, pp. 699–710.

33. Holroyd, E.A., Andrasik, F. and Westbrook, T. 'Cognitive Control of Tension Headaches'. *Cognitive Therapy Research* (1977), 1, pp. 121–33.

34. Paiva, T., Nunes, J.S., Moreira, A., Santos, J., Teixeira, J. and Barbosa, A. 'Effects of Frontalis EMG Biofeedback and Diazepam in the Treatment of Tension Headache'. *Headache* (1982), 22, pp. 216–20.

35. Sargent, J., Gree, E. and Walter, E. 'Preliminary Report on the Use of Autogenic Feedback Training in the Treatment of Migraine and Tension Headache'. *Psychosomatic Medicine* (1973), 35, pp. 129–35.

36. Blanchard, E.B., Theobald, D.E., Williamson, D.A., Silver, B.V. and Brown, D.A. 'Temperature Feedback in the Treatment of Migraine Headaches'. *Archives of General Psychiatry* (1978), 35, pp. 581–8.

37. Cohen, M.J., McArthur, D.L. and Rickles, W.H. 'Comparison of Four Biofeedback Treatments for Migraine Headaches: Physiological and Headache Variables'. *Psychosomatic Medicine* (1980), 42, pp. 463–80.

38. Friar, L.R. and Beatty, J.T. 'Migraine: Management by Operant Conditioning of Vasoconstriction'. *Journal of Consultant and Clinical Psychology* (1976), 44, pp. 46–53.

39. Knapp, T.H. 'Evidence of Sympathetic Deactivation by Temporal Vasoconstriction and Digital Vasoconstriction — Biofeedback in Migraine Patient'. *Headache* (1982), 22, pp. 233–6.

40. La Croix, J.M., Bock, J.C. and Lavis, S. 'Biofeedback and Relaxation in the Treatment of Migraine: Comparative Effectiveness and Physiological Correlates'. *Journal of Neurology, Neurosurgery and Psychiatry* (1983), 46, pp. 525–32.

41. Mitchell, K.R. and Mitchell, D.M. 'Migraine: An Exploratory Treatment Applications of Programmed Behaviour Therapy Techniques'. *Journal of Psychosomatic Research* (1971), 15, pp. 137–57.

42. Benson, H., Shapiro, D., Tursky, B. and Schwartz, G.E. 'Decreased Systolic Blood Pressure Through Operant Conditioning

Techniques in Patients with Essential Hypertension'. *Science* (1971), 173, pp. 740–2.

43. Elder, S.T., Ruiz, R., Deabler, H.L. and Dillenkoffer, R.L. 'Instrumental Conditioning of a Diastolic Blood Pressure in Essential Hypertensive Patients'. *Journal of Applied Behaviour Analysis* (1973), 6, pp. 377–82.

44. Kristt, D.A. and Engel, B.T. 'Learned Control of Blood Pressure in Patients with High Blood Pressure'. *Circulation* (1975), 51, pp. 370–8.

45. Steptoe, A. 'Blood Pressure Control: A Comparison of Feedback and Instructions Using Pulse Transit Time Feedback'. *Psychophysiology* (1976), 13, pp. 528–36.

46. Survit, R.S., Hager, J.L. and Feldman, T. 'The Role of Feedback in Voluntary Control of Blood Pressure Instructed Subjects'. *Journal of Applied Behaviour Analysis* (1977), 10, pp. 625–31.

47. Frankel, B.L., Patel, D.J., Horwitz, D., Friedwald, M.T. and Gaardner, K.P. 'Treatment of Hypertension with Biofeedback and Relaxation Techniques'. *Psychosomatic Medicine* (1978), 40, pp. 276–93.

48. Blanchard, E.R., Miller, S.R., Abel, C.C., Hayns, M.R. and Hicker, R. 'Evaluation of Biofeedback in the Treatment of Essential Hypertension'. *Journal of Applied Behaviour and Analysis* (1979), 12, pp. 99–110.

49. Fey, S.G. and Lindholm, E. 'Biofeedback and Progressive Relaxation: Effects on Systolic and Diastolic Blood Pressure and Heart Rate'. *Psychophysiology* (1978), 15, pp. 239–47.

50. Glasgow, M.S., Gaardner, K.R. and Engel, B.T. 'Behavioural Treatment of High Blood Pressure: II. Acute and Sustained Affects of Relaxation and Systolic Blood Pressure Biofeedback'. *Psychosomatic Medicine* (1982), 44, pp. 155–71.

51. McGrady, W.V., Yonker, R., Tan, S.Y., Fine, S.H. and Woewrner, M. 'The Effect of Biofeedback-assisted Relaxation on Blood Pressure and Selected Biochemical Parameters in Patients with Essential Hypertension'. *Biofeedback and Self-Regulation* (1981), 6, pp. 343–54.

52. Friedman, H. and Taub, H.A. 'The Use of Hypertension and Biofeedback Procedures for Essential Hypertension'. *International Journal of Clinical and Experimental Hypnosis* (1977), 25, pp. 335–47.

53. Patel, C. 'Yoga and Biofeedback in the Management of Hypertension'. *Lancet* (1973), 2, pp. 1053–5.

54. Patel, C. 'Twelve-month Follow-up of Yoga and Biofeedback in the Management of Hypertension'. *Lancet* (1975), 1, pp. 62–4.

55. Patel, C. and North, W.R.S. 'Randomised Controlled Trial of Yoga and Biofeedback in the Management of Hypertension'. *Lancet* (1975), 2, pp. 93–5.

56. Patel, C., Marmot, M.M. and Terry, D.J. 'Controlled Trial of Biofeedback-aided Behavioural Methods in Reducing Mild Hypertension'. *British Medical Journal* (1981), 282, pp. 2005–8.

57. Patel, C., Marmot, M.M., Terry, D.J., Carruthers, M., Hunt, B. and Patel, M. 'Trial of Relaxation in Reducing Coronary Risk: Four-year Follow-up'. *British Medical Journal* (1985), 290, pp. 1103–6.

58. Benson, H., Rosner, B.A., Marsetta, B.R. and Klemchuk, H.D.

'Decreased Blood Pressure in Pharmacologically Treated Hypertensive Patients Who Regularly Elicited the Relaxation Response'. *Lancet* (1974), 1, pp. 289–91.

59. Taylor, C.B., Farquhar, J.W., Nelson, E. and Agras, W.S. 'Relaxation Therapy and High Blood Pressure'. *Archives of General Psychiatry* (1977), 34, pp. 339–42.

60. Southam, M.A., Agra, W.S., Taylor, C.B. and Kraemer, H.C. 'Relaxation Training: Blood Pressure During Waking Day'. *Archives of General Psychiatry* (1982), 39, pp. 715–17.

61. Bali, L.R. 'Long-term Effect of Relaxation on Blood Pressure and Anxiety Levels in Essential Hypertensive Males. A Controlled Study'. *Psychosomatic Medicine* (1979), 41, pp. 637–46.

62. Irvine, M.J. 'A Controlled Study of Relaxation and Stress Management in the Treatment of Essential Hypertension'. DPhil thesis (Oxford University, Oxford, 1983).

63. Budsynski, T. 'Biofeedback Procedures in the Clinic'. *Seminars in Psychiatry* (1973), 5, pp. 537–47.

64. Raskin, M., Johnson, G. and Rondestvedt, J.H. 'Chronic Anxiety Treated by Feedback-induced Muscle Relaxation'. *Archives of General Psychiatry* (1973), 28, pp. 263–7.

65. Canter, A., Kondo, C.Y. and Knott, J.R. 'A Comparison of EMG Feedback and Progressive Muscle Relaxation Training in Anxiety Neurosis'. *British Journal of Psychiatry* (1975), 127, pp. 470–7.

66. Townsend, R.E., House, J.F. and Addario, D.A. 'A Comparison of Biofeedback-mediated Relaxation and Group Therapy in the Treatment of Chronic Anxiety'. *American Journal of Psychiatry* (1975), 132, pp. 598–601.

67. Hiebert, B.A. 'Comparison of EMG Feedback and Alternative Anxiety Treatment Programme'. *Biofeedback and Self-Regulation* (1981), 6, pp. 501–6.

68. Lavellee, Y.L., Lamontague, Y., Pinnard, G., Annable, L. and Tetreault, L. 'Effects of EMG Feedback, Diazepam and Their Combination on Chronic Anxiety'. *Journal of Psychosomatic Research* (1977), 21, pp. 65–71.

69. Porter, G. and Norris, P. *Why Me? Harnessing the Healing Power of the Human Spirit* (Stillpoint Publishing, Walpole, New Hampshire, 1985).

70. World Health Organization Collaboration Group. 'Multifactorial Trial in the Prevention of Coronary Heart Disease: III'. *European Heart Journal* (1983), 4, pp. 141–7.

USEFUL ADDRESSES

British Association for Holistic Health
Information Officer
179 Gloucester Place
London
NW1 6DX
Telephone: 01 262 5299

International Stress and Tension Control Association (UK Branch)
Information Officer
25 Sutherland Avenue
Leeds
LS8 1RY
Telephone: 0532 664260

Aleph One Ltd
The Old Courthouse
Bottisham
Cambridge
CB5 9BB
Telephone: 0223 811679

Biodata Limited
10 Stocks Street
Manchester
M8 8QG
Telephone: 061 834 6688

Further information on biofeedback instruments can be obtained from Aleph
One Ltd, address as above.

For courses in biofeedback therapy contact:

British Holistic Medical Association
179 Gloucester Place
London
NW1 6DX

British Postgraduate Medical Federation
33 Millman Street
London
WC1N 3EJ

APPENDIX: BIOFEEDBACK SERVICES IN BRITAIN

Most hospitals with a psychology department have some biofeedback equipment, as it is very widely used to help people with stress problems. It also is being used increasingly by physiotherapists for rehabilitation.

It is not usually possible to refer oneself for biofeedback treatment. A patient has to see his/her general practitioner who will refer the patient to the hospital. It is helpful if an initial enquiry is made to the psychology department as to whether they have equipment and people to use it, and if they are used to treating problems such as the patient's.

A few therapists offer biofeedback treatment privately. There is no system for licensing or training such therapists in Britain and no central register. A therapist may be found locally by contacting an organisation such as the British Association for Holistic Health or the International Stress and Tension Control Society or a supplier of equipment such a Aleph One Ltd or Biodata Ltd (see above). In any case it should be established that a therapist has experience with referent problems, and names of satisfied clients supplied if in doubt.

Because biofeedback instruments do not change patients, but only give them information they can use to change themselves, they are intrinsically safe and unlikely to cause harm. They are therefore sold to the general public, at prices from about £35 upwards. Suppliers should provide good instructions and advice on the application of their products to particular cases.

12

Hypnosis

Jacques Tamin

INTRODUCTION

Hypnosis has been likened to the feeling you get just before falling asleep. Yet it is far from being 'sleep' (*hypnos* in Greek), so 'hypnosis' is a very misleading term. Indeed, it is not even a state of relaxation, though relaxation is often used as part of hypnotherapy. In fact, it can sometimes be quite the opposite — a feeling of intense concentration.

Fulder,[1] in his description of hypnosis, suggests that it is '. . . a state in which (a) the cognitive controls over the mind are loosened or dissociated; and (b) the person is not asleep and can receive and act on messages, is a hypnotic or partially hypnotic state'.

Hypnosis, or hypnotherapy in the context of health care, can be described as the deliberate use of the 'trance state'.

We all go in and out of trance several times a day, usually without realising that we are doing so. When you can recall your last holiday with such vivid detail that it is almost as though you were there again, you are in a 'trance'. Every time you can see yourself, in your 'mind's eye', acting out some of your past or future, you are in trance. Each time your mind 'escapes' from a boring lecture by 'floating away', once again, that is trance!

Trance is an altered state of consciousness. Before looking at what this means exactly, and at the practical applications, we will see how hypnosis was 'discovered'.

HISTORICAL BACKGROUND

Hypnosis has probably been used for therapeutic purposes throughout history, both knowingly and unknowingly. From the primitive tribes and their 'witch doctors' to oriental techniques such as yoga, a trance state has been the means through which 'cures' have been effected.

The western discovery of hypnosis began with Franz Mesmer in 1773. His theory, however, was that some sort of 'fluid' was redistributed by the force of 'animal magnetism'. He could effect 'cures' on neurotic patients, in an atmosphere of mystical theatricals. However, his contemporaries disproved the scientific basis of his theory, and he was largely discredited.

In the 19th century, several physicians revived some interest in the technique. Among them was James Braid, an English physician who coined the term 'hypnosis' and stated that it occurred due to suggestion. But when Freud used hypnosis, he found its cures too superficial for his purposes; his rejection of the technique was a major setback in the development of hypnosis.

During the First World War, Ernst Simmel, a German psychoanalyst developed a technique he called hypnoanalysis for the treatment of war neuroses. Work with hypnosis during both world wars to treat such conditions received a lot of interest in the United States.

Most of the recent developments have come from the United States, and such men as Milton Erickson (1901–80) and Herbert Spiegel have largely influenced the current practice of hypnosis.

PRESENT CONCEPTS OF HYPNOSIS

Hypnosis focuses on the premise that each individual has much more innate ability than he/she ever believes is possible. Whether we choose to ignore that ability or to use it constructively is only up to us.

Contrary to popular belief, the therapist does not 'do' anything to the patient. The patient does it to himself/herself. This intrinsic ability, and the ability to learn about one's innate potential and improve it was stressed by both Erickson and Spiegel. More recent research using controlled hypnosis experiments have demonstrated an ability to control pain tolerance, reduce response to superficial burns and control blood pressure.[2,3]

These studies illustrate the potential within each one of us to exert much more control over our bodies, for example in alleviating pain, and over the mind, for example in improving concentration or memory. However, a hypnotherapist can only teach and guide one to use one's own 'power'.

THE CONSCIOUS AND SUBCONSCIOUS MIND

Our minds work on two levels — conscious and subconscious. We are aware of what goes on in our conscious mind, but not always so of our subconscious one. Yet the latter is possibly more powerful and can certainly affect our physical and mental health very dramatically. However, it basically wants the same result as our conscious mind, that is, our safety and happiness. When the conscious and unconscious minds work independently, conflict can arise which may be physically or psychologically detrimental to our state of health.

For example, at some point in one's career one may decide to work much harder to gain some advancement. The subconscious mind, however, may find that you are doing too much, and to 'protect' you, may make you feel increasingly tired. Thus, the harder one consciously tries, the harder it is to do the work. This gives rise to increasing feelings of frustration, stress and tension, and ultimately wears you out even more! If, on the other hand, your conscious and subconscious minds had understood what each was trying to do, they could have reached a compromise, and avoided internal conflict. Trance can allow these two parts of your mind to communicate in order to prevent or resolve such problems.

THERAPEUTIC APPLICATIONS

There is a wide range of possible applications of hypnosis. Which therapeutic aspect one chooses to study may be influenced by one's existing nursing specialty.

Midwifery

For example, during pregnancy hypnosis has been found to be useful and enjoyable, both antenatally and postnatally, and during labour. This would be an ideal technique for midwives since they may already have a first-hand knowledge of trance, which occurs regularly during their antenatal relaxation classes (however, they may not recognise a light trance, unless they have been trained in hypnosis). Furthermore, their expertise in the process of labour as a natural event, and their understanding of the fears and myths that surround labour, provide a sound formation from which to specialise in hypnotherapy. During antenatal hypnosis, the understanding of how her body works and what happens during labour is received at a deeper and more personal level by each pregnant woman, and as with many therapies, emphasis is placed upon individual care and support according to each person's needs.

Accident and emergency

Hypnosis also offers considerable benefits in casualty departments, where for example the casualty nurse could allay the anxieties of a frightened child quickly and easily rather than having to forcefully smother the blanket-wrapped child howling its head off. Prior to suturing or taking blood, it is possible to put the child into a quick trance, perform the procedure and have the child go away with a smile. And a relieved mother usually looks on in amazement! As a practising physician, I have found this technique infinitely more rewarding and less physically and emotionally stressful for the patient, relatives and staff concerned.

Dental hypnosis

An increasing number of dentists use hypnosis to treat dental pains, and other related problems such as fear of dentists and needle phobias.[4] Moreover, some who are also adept and experienced in hypnotherapy also treat many medical and psychological conditions. There is no reason for those who were particularly adept at hypnotherapy not to treat some conditions outside that sphere. In doing so, practitioners would be able to generate a more holistic rather than symptomatic approach to health care.

Other problems that are commonly treated with hypnosis can be listed as follows:

(1) Mainly physical: migraine, dysmenorrhoea (painful periods), intractable pain (hopefully after a diagnosis has been made), asthma.
(2) Mainly psychological: anxiety states, phobias — such as fear of

flying, insects or thunder, depression (this is controversial, as will be seen later).

(3) Childhood disorders: tics, stammers, bedwetting, nailbiting.

(4) Behavioural problems: cigarette smoking, overeating.

MISCONCEPTIONS ABOUT HYPNOSIS

There are many myths and misconceptions about hypnosis, which you would be wise to dispel fairly early on. The main ones are the following:

Hypnosis involves magical or mystical forces

Your patient should understand that the power for self-improvement comes from within himself/herself, and not you or any 'external forces'. You are there only to teach him/her about the potential he/she already has, and to guide in its use to help with a particular problem.

Hypnosis is sleep

It has nothing to do with sleep, and the client will definitely be wide awake. Occasionally, a patient does fall asleep when relaxing deeply, but that is not a trance state. One has to wait for the client to wake up so that there may be interchange of information. The word 'sleep' meaning a trance state is still used by some therapists, but this can be confusing for the patient and is best avoided. Some patients will tell you that they are 'hyper aware' of everything that goes on around them, while others become less aware, maybe focusing only on your voice or their experience. Both are equally valid experiences of trance and can be used effectively for therapy. Patients can feel deeply relaxed or be in intense concentration, but should be receptive to your voice, ideas, suggestions and explanations. And they cannot do this if they are asleep!

The patient is under your control

The misconception that the patient will be under your control and unable to resist your 'commands' is quite wrong — even in deepest trance, our moral values and beliefs do not change. I therefore reassure patients that if they objected to or disagreed with anything I said while they were in trance, they would simply reject this, or come out of trance if they wished to. They will accept suggestions only because they realise that it is for their own good; but they may also accept a suggestion such as feeling their hand becoming lighter because it is part of learning to improve their own trance. On no account would a therapist make suggestions just to make a fool of a patient. Such 'therapists' would have no place in conventional therapy, let alone in hypnotherapy!

Stage hypnosis

There is still a popular uninformed image of the hypnotist saying: 'you *will* do . . .', and the subject, unable to resist, obeying every command. Many of us have seen this on some stage or other. Why then does this happen? First, these performers are very skilled hypnotists. But their main skill is in *choosing* their subjects. Only those who would really like to play the fool in public would accept these suggestions; they have their glorious moment of exhibitionism without having to take responsibility for it.

Good hypnotic subjects have 'weaker' minds

The popular concept here is that the 'stronger-willed' hypnotist imposes his thoughts on 'weaker-minded' subjects. So you will often hear: 'I can't be hypnotised. I'm very strong-willed.' You can explain that this is an attribute that can help in the use of trance. In effect subjects are learning to control their own minds *with* their own minds. So the more intelligent, the more purposeful, the more 'with it' they are, the better and more effective they will be in learning about this form of self-control.

Indeed, the only definitely non-hypnotisable group are the mentally subnormal. Schizophrenics form another group who find it difficult to maintain sufficient concentration, but very skilled therapists are able to match their reality, and thus communicate with them. (Such techniques are beyond the scope of this book, but suggestions for further reading are given at the end of this chapter, p. 201). Otherwise, most of the normal population have the ability to go into trance, therapists with a vast amount of experience admit that they have yet to meet someone unable to do so.

Hypnosis is dangerous or harmful

If hypnotherapy has one overriding advantage over conventional medicine, it is its lack of side-effects. In fact the only type of side-effect (if it can be called that) caused by treatment with hypnosis is a general feeling of wellbeing and an increased positiveness about oneself. This warm 'glow' one feels after experiencing trance tends to occur whatever was the original reason for learning about trance.

Going in and out of trance is very safe and beneficial. When this trance is also being used to treat a particular problem, it is reasonable to expect the therapist, the guide, to be familiar with that condition. One should not expect a therapist who knows nothing about depression to start treating depressed patients. In this respect, any attempt at therapy, or advice, could be inappropriate whether using trance or not.

So long as hypnotherapy is used in a responsible way, there is no risk at all to the patient. One must expect all potential therapists to undergo adequate training and be familiar with the fields where they expect to use hypnotherapy. As mentioned before, some will progress and expand their areas of expertise.

BASIC TECHNIQUES OF HYPNOSIS

A simple conventional technique is described here, to illustrate the different facets of treatment using the trance state. However, bear in mind that there are wide variations, and experienced therapists will omit some stages or take them in a different order depending on the situation.

Conventionally, hypnotherapy is broken down into the following states: trance induction, deepening, ego strengthening, post-hypnotic suggestions, ending the trance state.

Trance induction

Trance can be formally started by a recognisable signal such as asking the patient to fix a point until his eyes feel heavy and want to close. This 'eye closure' is then taken to be a sign of entry into trance. This description is an oversimplification of the dynamics of the situation, and can be considered as only a beginner's guide to trance.

Deepening

The patient may want to go deeper into trance. You can help him/her to achieve this by progressive relaxation, which is a gradual relaxing of the various muscle groups of the body.

In conjunction with this it is possible to use distraction techniques such as counting backwards, subtracting a number repeatedly from 100, or any fairly simple calculation you can think of. This has the effect of forcing the conscious mind to focus on this task, making it easier for the subconscious mind to 'rise to the surface'.

Following this, arm levitation, arm rigidity, or feelings of heat or cold may be suggested to allow the patient to slip into deeper and deeper trance. Suggestions can be made where the patient imagines going down a lift or a tunnel, sinking deeper into the subconscious mind while doing so.

Alternatively, one can suggest that he/she may wish to imagine being on a beach, or taking a walk down a country lane, and the more vivid the colours, smells, sounds and sensations become, the deeper the trance.

There are a multitude of such deepening techniques, which may be used in any order, or none at all, if this is felt to be more appropriate.

When training in hypnosis it would be wise to try most of these techniques gradually, and find out for yourself which suit you best. It is important, however, not to be too standardised in approach, as each patient is unique. Once you have gained some experience, the aim should be to develop a range of techniques with which you feel comfortable, thus making it possible to offer the patient the route into deeper trance which they find easiest and most enjoyable.

Ego strengthening

At this stage, the patient will be at some level of trance, and more receptive to suggestions. In ego strengthening, a spectrum of positive suggestions are offered for the subconscious mind to choose from and act upon.

For example, the therapist may suggest that physically they will be fitter, more relaxed, feel better about themselves. Mentally, they will learn how to recognise their inner strength, and be able to use it when desired. This will enhance feelings of self-assurance and independence, and self-confidence will grow.

As these are basic truths, the patient will be able to make these suggestions come true if they wish to. Emphasis can be placed upon a particular area that is a special problem. For example, if there is a fear of going far from home, the therapist may suggest: 'as you become more and more in touch with yourself, and more and more in control of yourself, you will find it easier to feel more and more independent, self-assured, confident, in control, at peace with yourself, whatever the external surroundings . . .'

Even if you were to use the same wording for this ego boosting to all your patients, it is surprising how personal this message feels in trance. This is because the subconscious mind is able to select the part that is specially appropriate for it.

Post-hypnotic suggestions

In the therapeutic setting, post-hypnotic suggestions are used to reinforce the learning that has gone on during trance.

A typical post-hypnotic suggestion would be that the patient would continue to feel better day by day, would understand himself/herself better and use his/her potential more effectively.

If the patient had been taught auto-hypnosis or self-hypnosis, the suggestion could be that he/she would enjoy using the technique regularly, finding it easier and easier to do, and also be able to achieve even deeper trance if he/she so wished.

Post-hypnotic suggestions, as other suggestions, will work only if the patient accepts them. Where the patient does want to get better, these suggestions will work very powerfully indeed.

Ending the trance state

Often the therapist will do this by counting slowly, asking the patient to lighten the trance slowly until he/she comes out of it.

Personally, I usually tell my patients: 'When you are ready to come out of trance, make it become lighter and lighter until you are out of trance, feeling fully refreshed and wide awake, with all the normal sensations returning to every part of your body.'

In this way, patients are aware that they are controlling their own trances, and will eventually be able to do this on their own.

OTHER TECHNIQUES OF HYPNOSIS

There is a wide variety of possible techniques, because of the range of conditions that can be treated with hypnosis, and the uniqueness of each individual. Here are a few examples to illustrate this.

For example, with children in an outpatient department one could ask them about their television programme or their favourite game. Then ask: 'Do you want to see that show or play that game. Yes? Then close your eyes, switch the TV set on, and see that show. (Or hold your doll, do you want to comb her hair, etc.). While you watch (or play), just feel comfortable, drowsy and dreamy.' Of course, you have to say this in a reassuring, comforting manner, but basically that is all the level of trance you need for taking blood or suturing.

If a deeper trance is needed, they will usually cooperate readily with such suggestions as: 'See a large red balloon in front of you. See it rise, slowly and gently. It has a piece of string tied to your right wrist. Feel the tug on it as it rises. Up and up it goes, higher and higher and higher . . . .' And soon you see the hand rising.

Ego boosting should include feelings of security and being loved. The child should look forward to becoming stronger and have a special 'power' to do some special things.

Tics and stammers

Children who stammer can be taught to relax the muscles of their mouth by clenching a fist. Gradually they will learn to stammer less and less, both in and out of trance. This is similar for tics — I ask them to start their muscles twitching in trance until they feel they cannot stop it. Then with the fist-clenching technique, allow these muscles to relax and stop twitching. Again, they do this several times in and out of trance.

After this first session, they practise this regularly, two or three times a day, through self-hypnosis. They quickly learn that they can control this symptom, and more importantly, that they can gain some control in improving themselves. Subsequent sessions mainly reinforce this learning.

It is possible to teach any patient 'waking trance', once he/she is sufficiently familiar with the trance state. This involves the patient having his/her eyes open, and responding normally to the ouside world, but actualy being in trance. This is useful if, say, the patient suffers from panic attacks, and would usually have tried to run away from the situation. By using a practised signal, like pressing two fingers together, he/she can achieve enough self-control to over-come these feelings. Another use of the same technique is in migraine sufferers, who can abort an attack and continue with their daily activities.

A very elegant and quick form of self-hypnosis has been developed by Spiegel (see further reading, p. 201).

Conversational hypnosis

Other advanced techniques include 'conversational hypnosis', where there is no formal trance induction, and the patient may not even be aware that he/she is in trance. It is also possible to use your own trance to induce your patient's. For example, I sometimes induce anaesthesia in the back of one hand, and pass a hypodermic needle through. (*Note:* Such procedures should only be attempted following qualified courses in hypnosis, strictly ensuring the sterility of all equipment.) Often the patient would be in deep trance just watching this, so I would say 'Right, now let yourself slip deeper and deeper within your own mind . . .', and continue treatment from this deep trance. There are other non-verbal methods of trance induction, but they are all best seen demonstrated by an experienced therapist.

THERAPEUTIC STRATEGIES

This is the part the beginner finds difficult. As you now know, it is easy to slip into trance. We can all do it. But once the patient is in trance, the beginner thinks 'what now?'

Let us illustrate the problem by considering a phobia, for example a fear of spiders. Most patients may need only relatively light trance to learn to relax effectively and consistently. Then in light trance they may be progressively desensitised. The benefits of this learning are generally complete and lifelong, and there is no recurrence.

A small proportion, however, may fail at this relatively super-ficial approach. When more advanced techniques such as age regres-sion are used, it may emerge that they had a terrible fright from a spider (real, toy or picture) at the age of four, but had subsequently forgotten that episode. But once the episode is relived and dealt with appropriately, the problem disappears.

A smaller proportion still may not be cured. With deeper analysis and regression, the phobia may not relate to spiders at all — for example, it may be due to a deep feeling of insecurity from early childhood, partly because of misunderstanding their parents' attitudes. When this is redressed, they lose their phobia forever.

GENERAL RULES IN HYPNOSIS

The simple techniques should be attempted initially. Not all your patients need deep hypnoanalysis or age regressing! Do not attempt to provide answers or solutions. Your patients have the correct answers within themselves. The therapist's aim is to guide them there, first by improving their self-understanding, then by allowing them to realise that they have more than one course of action to choose from. They should be taught to see their problems in perspective, within the overall 'positiveness' that their life can be, in order to cope with new problems much more effectively.

The best predictor of therapeutic success is your patient's motivation and not the ability to slip into trance easily, or even depth of trance he/she reaches. Therapy involves a conscious cooperation between the patient and therapist, and a lot of hard work on their part. Hypnotherapy should never be the 'easy way out', and it never is. Because of that, it is important to give the patient the credit for any self-improvement. Unlike conventional therapy, the patient is responsible for his health and wellbeing, and this responsibility involves the setbacks as well as the rewards.

CONCLUSIONS

The ability to use trance positively and constructively is exciting and challenging. Yet it is a technique we all could use with great ease.

The therapeutic potential of using trance is wide-ranging and free from side-effects. It also gives patients the chance to learn about their personal inner strength, to understand themselves better and to cope with new problems with a fresh outlook.

And most important of all, hypnotherapy has returned the responsibility for healing to the patient — a responsibility that conventional medicine has denied for too long.

REFERENCES

1. Fulder, S. *The Handbook of Complementary Medicine* (Coronet Books, London, 1984), p. 192.
2. Chapman, L.F., Goodell, H. and Wolff, H.G. 'Changes in Tissue Vulnerability Induced during Hypnotic Suggestion', *Journal of Psychosomatic Research* (1959), 4, pp. 99-105.
3. Maslach, C., Marshall, G. and Zimbardo, P.G. 'Hypnotic Control of Peripheral Skin Temperature: A Case Report. *Psychophysiology* (1972), 9, pp. 600-5.
4. Hartland, J. *Medical and Dental Hypnosis* (Baillière Tindall, London, 1971).

BIBLIOGRAPHY AND FURTHER READING

The following are books for those who would like to learn more about hypnotherapy. They are not all as easy for the inexperienced to read, so there are also notes on what to expect.

Bandler, R. *Using Your Brain — For a Change*. (Utah, Real People Press, 1985). A very readable and illuminating book. It assumes prior knowledge of trance techniques, but provides a positive approach to direct change.

Erickson, M.H., Hershman, S. and Secter, I.I. *The Practical Application of Medical and Dental Hypnosis*. (Chicago, Chicago Seminars on Hypnosis Publishing Co., 1981). A good basic book, with wide scope and the correct modern philosophy of hypnosis.

Rosen, S. (ed.) *My Voice Will Go With You: The Teaching Tales of Milton H. Erickson*. (W.W. Norton, London, New York, 1982). Very readable. Provides a fascinating insight into the way this modern 'guru' of hypnotherapy used to practise, but does not provide the basic grounding in techniques. An eventual 'must' for those who will do analytical work.

Spiegel, H. and Spiegel, D. *Trance and Treatment: Clinical Uses of Hypnosis*. (Basic Books Inc., New York, 1978). A very interesting book, but harder to follow. It includes a description of Spiegel's hypnotic induction profile — a standardised clinical test for trance capacity. Overall a more scientific and rigorous approach to the subject.

USEFUL ADDRESSES

Mrs M. Samuels
BSMDH
42 Links Rd
Ashstead
Surrey
KT21 2HJ

The Secretary
Manchester School of Hypnosis
36 St Bee's Close
Denmark Rd
Manchester
M14 4GG

APPENDIX: COURSES IN HYPNOSIS

If you wish to learn more about hypnosis, it is advisable to attend a course with reputable teachers.

The British Society for Medical and Dental Hypnosis run excellent courses for doctors and dentists at basic, intermediate and advanced levels. There are a few places offered to medical students, but unfortunately, not to other health care professionals.

Courses aimed specifically for nurses and midwives are run by the Manchester School of Hypnosis, who also run courses for doctors and medical students. Other health care professionals may be admitted; please enquire at the address above.

13

Social Skills

Jean Orr

INTRODUCTION

Within the range of complementary therapies it could be argued that there is a common emphasis on communicating with the client in a way that helps the therapeutic process. Unlike much of conventional medicine and health care, the interaction between the therapist and client is part of any treatment and can make that treatment more effective. Therefore a knowledge of social skills will be useful to everyone whether involved in complementary therapies or practising orthodox health care, and will help them to understand the clients' needs and to be aware of the messages that they as therapists may be presenting to clients.

All of us communicate at some level with the world around us. We have learnt through growing up to ask questions, to listen to people, to make appropriate gestures, to understand non-verbal communication, and to keep a conversation going. But do we communicate as well as we could? Increasingly, it is recognised that these skills can be identified, broken down into measurable components, and can therefore be studied and learnt. We are probably aware of interviewers who put people at ease, ask interesting questions and get the best out of the situation. We also can probably think of those who are bad communicators and who make us feel uncomfortable in their presence. This may be because they come too close to us, or do not show interest, or do not appear to listen to what we say.

FEATURES OF SOCIAL SKILLS

A socially skilled person will possess the ability to behave in an appropriate manner in any given situation. According to Hargie, Saunders and Dickson,[1] a social skill is 'a set of goal directed interrelated social behaviours which can be learned and which are under the control of the individual'. There are five main features of social skills.

(1) Socially skilled behaviours are goal-directed. This means the skills are used for some purpose to achieve an outcome. For example, if we wish to indicate that we are listening to someone we may sit forward in the chair, maintain eye contact, nod and say 'yes, I see'.
(2) Socially skilled behaviours should be interrelated in order to achieve a goal. As in the example above, more than one skill is being used and the skills are used together for maximum effect.
(3) Social skills are defined in terms of identifiable units of behaviour, so that within a main skill such as questioning the interviewer is using non-verbal skills such as head nods, eye contact and listening.
(4) Social skills can be learned. Children learn how to behave by modelling themselves on adults or peers and by imitating what they see. They also learn by having their behaviour reinforced or rewarded so that they will develop the skills which gain most praise.
(5) Social skills should be under the control of the individual. Probably we have ways of behaving which are annoying or distracting and these can be identified and changed. For example, if there are individuals who tend to come too close when talking to us and make us feel uncomfortable, that individual can be helped to identify this trait and can learn a different pattern of behaviour.

The nurse cannot remain outside or separate from the relationship with the individual patient/client. This relationship is not a static entity nor does it have clearly defined boundaries. There are contradictions, ambiguities and conflicts within the relationship and roles are being constantly renegotiated. The interaction has the features of any coming together of two people, it is affected by both participants and both participants are affected by it. The type of relationship has two elements, the observed and the observer, the known and the unknown, but it is the very act of the observing that the observer becomes the observed, the unknown becomes the known. The fluidity of the interaction belies the traditional image of the client/professional relationship in which the professional conducts an interview without deviating from the aims, being side-tracked by the client or being asked direct questions about their personal life. There is an assumption that the client will act in a way which is acceptable and to ensure this, professionals have an investment in defining the way things are.[2] This definition is reflected in the kind of services traditionally offered, to whom they are offered and what methods of service delivery are employed. In essence the professional's concept of the client's problems shapes what the professional believes is needed. This is, of course, within a fairly limited perspective because professionals define client needs by professional skills.

The relationship between nurse and client is significant in that the nurse utilises it as part of the therapeutic process. The nurse needs to develop a relationship so she can collect data to identify problems and needs, formulate a plan of action and set both short-term and long-term goals with the client's consent. Within the field of alternative health strategies the nurse must move away from a didactic model of 'being in charge' and telling the patient what to do to a partnership based on trust and reciprocity. Within this partnership there is a mutual learning experience in that the nurse learns from the client and with the client as they explore the client's problems and lifestyle.[3] Rather than the nurse being the 'expert', the client is seen to be the expert on his/her own life and experience. Within the relationship there is respect for different values, and the uniqueness of each individual is observed and respected. The nurse then cannot force anything on the client if such a relationship exists, but must recognise that often the client will have different standards which must be respected and observed.

The relationship is seen as a therapeutic one and as such is the vehicle for employing strategies which will lead to the achievement of defined goals, and it will be seen to facilitate the feeling of trust between nurse and client. Trust is defined by Wiedenback and Falls[4] as 'the connection that exists between two people who are in close contact with one another, and have a firm belief in each other's honesty, reliability and accountability'. It may be said, then, that trust is the foundation upon which effective care is built, and is necessary in a relationship if nurse and client are to work together and follow a problem-solving process. It is the therapeutic relationship which

205

facilitates the growth and strengthening of this trust between the nurse and client.

NON-VERBAL COMMUNICATION

This term is used to describe all forms of human communication that are not controlled by speech. There are however, non-verbal aspects of speech which are called paralanguage, and this denotes the way meaning can be communicated by the tone of voice, the speed and pitch. For example, saying 'I really enjoyed that meal' in a flat clipped tone will have a different meaning than when said with emphasis and variety in tone.

The term paralanguage also covers the sounds made which have meaning but are not words. For example, 'mm-hmm' 'aha' 'uh huh' are frequently used in order to convey the fact we are listening without actually saying words.[1]

Information sent out and received about the people we meet involves a wide range of non-verbal communication. This can be illustrated by imagining meeting a client for the first time — try to think about the information gained by looking at them.

First, an impression of their dress and appearance will be gained. Are they untidy or ill-kempt, are they formally or casually dressed, are they wearing badges that say something about their political beliefs and do they look well cared for. Conclusions can often be drawn (rightly or wrongly) about appearance; for example if someone is dressed in a punk style it could be interpreted that they are deviant drug-takers. While appearance will imply something about the person, it is important to be aware that our own subjective value judgements could cause unfair labelling or stereotyping.

Second, an impression of the mood of clients can be gained by the way they hold their body. Clients who are anxious may show this by clenching their hands, pulling at clothing, adjusting their hair; they may have difficulty sitting still and may frown, bite their lips or show other nervous movements such as fiddling with a pen or watch. On the other hand a client who is depressed may sit slumped in a chair, looking downcast and refusing to respond to conversation. The skilled nurse will be able to tell the mood of the patient from the non-verbal behaviour, and therefore respond to these cues.

The range of information received by non-verbal communication is probably more than is generally acknowledged.[5] Part of being an effective nurse is to interpret these messages as a vital element of assessment and therapy. Equally, nurses tell clients more than they wish to admit about themselves. Nurses should be sensitive to these aspects of non-verbal communication by recognising that even before they speak they have conveyed messages to patients that will have a fundamental impact on the interaction.

An important aspect of non-verbal communication is that it can contradict the spoken word. Clients may be saying 'No' and nodding their heads to mean 'Yes', or saying 'I want to do this' but shaking their heads to mean 'No'. Clients might be saying 'I feel fine' when their bodies implies that they are tense and anxious. There often can be discrepancies between a person's eyes and mouth so that they smile with their mouth but not their eyes. When contradictory messages are being given, it is the non-verbal messages which are said to be telling the truth.[6]

Types of non-verbal communication

Bodily contact

It is through bodily contact that a large range of meaning is expressed, from the close proximity of lovers to the fleeting contact of shaking hands with a stranger. Bodily contact is governed by many social rules and can vary considerably between cultures.[7] For example, the French often kiss each other, and in some countries such as Turkey, men kiss each other and walk with their arms round each other, but in Britain this would not be seen as appropriate behaviour. Within nursing, touching people is interpreted as part of the usual course of work in order to carry out treatments. However touch is also important when conveying encouragement, concern and emotional support in patient care. When used in a therapeutic way touch can help in reducing clients' distress or anxiety, or where there is difficulty in articulating feelings.

In these situations it is useful to make contact with the client by, for example, touching his/her arm, taking his/her hand, or putting an arm round his/her shoulder in order to convey concern and empathy. This practice is often avoided or interpreted as 'un-professional' in some way. However, when a client is distressed, touch may be enough to convey a message of concern through our body language.[8] The nurse should, however, be aware that a client may sometimes be distressed by touch if it is sexually threatening, or if the client has unpleasant memories of being touched. For example, a woman who has been sexually assaulted or harassed may be distressed by bodily contact especially if the nurse is a man. In such a case, it may be necessary to ask the client if it is all right to touch her. By carefully observing the non-verbal body language the nurse can respond in an appropriate manner.

Orientation

It is not only important to be aware of the distance between oneself and the patient, but also to realise that the physical position adopted will affect the relationship. To sit side by side is seen as a cooperative position whereas to sit opposite someone implies competitiveness. For conversation or consultation it is best to sit at a 90° angle preferably with no desks or barriers in between. It is also counterproductive to be at a different height from the patient, as to be higher is seen as 'superior'.[9] Patients in bed frequently experience this when doctors and nurses tower over them often from the end of the bed. This is not conducive to good interaction; it is better to sit at the same level as the patients or even a little lower so that the patient can feel superior or at least equal.

Personal space

Underpinning much of the non-verbal aspects of communication is the concept of personal space. This may be interpreted as the 'area' each person has immediately surrounding his/her body and which is disturbing to him/her if other people enter this space. The area is like an egg shape with the pointed end in front of the person.[1]

An example of this can be observed on a crowded tube or bus: when standing close to a stranger individuals may try to turn aside, avoid eye contact or quickly glance away. Bags or briefcases may be held in front of the body to form a barrier. At parties people may be observed defending their personal space with a glass or plate or folded arms.

It is important to avoid moving too close to clients as it may make them back away or become tense. When you are about to invade a client's personal space it is best to say what you are going to do, make contact on the shoulder or arm, and avoid sudden movements such as pulling off bedclothes or clothing.[8] This is particularly important when touching sexually sensitive areas, such as breasts or genitals, or where there is an old injury or disfigurement.

Personal territory

While personal space is the immediate area surrounding a person, personal territory refers to the wider area in which a person seeks to establish a sense of intimacy and belonging.[9] All individuals seek to establish personal territory, whether at home or at work where, for example, an office may be arranged in a way that implies a sense of security. Some people may feel it necessary to defend their territory by having a desk between them and others, while teachers may feel most comfortable distancing themselves from pupils behind a table or rostrum.

In defending personal territory in this way barriers are set up which hinder effective communication and interaction. For example, a teacher would achieve considerably more participation with students in a circle and no desks. When visiting clients in their own home it is necessary to be aware of their personal territory. It might be seen as threatening by some clients when health or social workers make a visit, particularly if the visitor appears to be judgemental or officious and does not respect the client's privacy.

Proximity

Proximity is how close people are to each other. As individuals we tend to respond to an invisible line between ourselves and others; if we are too far away the other person may feel inaccessible and the interaction will be ineffectual, if too close, then the other person can feel uncomfortable and may try to move away.[10] It is important to realise that people can have differing optimum distances and what is too close for one person may cause another to feel insecure. Individuals also interact at a closer distance to people when standing rather than sitting.

A sitting distance of 1.5–1.8 m (5–6 feet) is common for work situations but 2.4–3.0 m (8–10 feet) seems to be an acceptable distance in a person's home. When standing, the normal space is about 0.9–1.2 m (3–4 feet).[11] It is helpful to acknowledge that proximity is related to status; thus the higher status a person feels, the more relaxed they may feel to approach a lower status person — but not vice versa. For example, a supervisor may feel able to stand closer to a worker than a worker feels comfortable when in close proximity to the supervisor. We see this in professional relationships where the professional takes up the position closer to the patient than would be appropriate in normal interaction.

The notion of personal distance has been classified by Hall[12] into four main zones depending on the purpose of the interaction.

Intimate zone. Those who have an intimate relationship with each other will interact at a distance of about 45 cm (18 inches).

Personal zone. In a close personal relationship the normal distance is 45 cm (18 inches) to 1.2 m (4 feet).

Social/consultative zone. In professional interaction the normal distance is 2.7 to 3.6 m (9 to 12 feet).

Public zone. Speakers at public lectures are usually at a distance of over 3.6 m (12 feet) from the audience.

However it is notable that these may vary in different cultures, and staff should be aware of the impact social distancing may have during interaction.

Facial expression

Much can be learnt from clients' facial expression and conversely clients learn what staff are feeling and thinking. Our language is full of statements such as 'she couldn't face me', 'his face was a picture', 'it was written all over his face'. These everyday comments imply the values many people ascribe to facial expression when interpreting those such as anger, guilt, fear, joy, etc. The eyes and mouth are probably the two main areas of the face that convey expression and may indeed convey contradictory messages.[13] For example, one may smile with the mouth but not the eyes, or look interested with the eyes but be stifling a yawn. Clients will often demonstrate anxiety, fear or embarrassment by facial expression while saying all is well, and in such cases it is the facial expression that has most credence.[14]

Eye contact

Throughout language and literature there are many references to the importance we place on eye contact (for example, 'he couldn't look me in the eye', 'eyes are the windows of the soul', 'he is shifty-eyed'). The more intimate we are, or the more trust we place in a person, the more eye contact we tend to have.

Although we may not be aware of it there are social 'rules' governing eye contact; for example, the speaker will look away from the listener for part of the time when speaking, but will establish direct eye contact from time to time to check out that she/he is being heard.[6,9] Frequently when the speaker is concentrating on what he/she is saying, eye contact may be minimal, whereas towards the end of conversation, eye contact is more frequent. This acts as a signal for the listener to respond or to start speaking. If the speaker does not establish some eye contact it may mean that he/she is distressed or uncomfortable about what is being said. If something unpleasant is about to be expressed to a patient there is a tendency to avoid eye contact, or staff may appear to be looking at notes or helping the patient on with clothes, etc. It would seem that it is very difficult to maintain conversation when the listener does not look at the speaker, and even the most articulate and talkative people cease talking in the absence of any response.[15]

When a client is talking it is valuable to demonstrate clearly that one is listening by appropriate eye contact. In this context 'appropriate' eye contact also reflects the social mores of communication. Excessive eye contact may be interpreted as threatening. You may have heard people in potentially violent situations saying 'what are you staring at?'. There is a status difference in eye contact, those of higher status maintaining greater eye contact than those of lower status.[16] This does, however, vary between the sexes with women being expected to 'lower their eyes', particularly in the Asian culture, and this may pose problems for a female nurse working with Asian male patients or colleagues as her behaviour may be seen as aggressive.[17]

The appropriate use of eye contact is most important during interaction but there are situations when eye contact may feel uncomfortable. In these cases it seems better to focus on a point just above the bridge of the nose. This gives the impression of eye contact but is easier to maintain in situations which the nurse finds difficult.

Hand and head movements

Body movements also play an important part in giving messages. Fidgeting hands and clenched fists show a person's mood. Gestures which denote anxiety include playing with hair, rubbing the face, fiddling with a pen or watch or tapping the feet. A wide range of gestures have acquired meaning in our society, but again these are not the same for all cultures.[18]

Just as we pick up messages about the client, so they can tell things about us. If we strongly disapprove of what a client is saying there may be a tendency to draw back, fold our arms or find an excuse to get up and move away. In this respect it may be necessary to assess realistically our own body movements which may have become habits, and try to change behaviour which may be distracting or revealing.

VERBAL COMMUNICATION

Nurses may experience difficulties in communicating with clients and these can be as a result of the following factors:

(1) differences in social class which may be obvious in dress, accent, language or mannerisms;
(2) differences in ethnic background;
(3) differences in cultural or religious beliefs;
(4) differences in values;
(5) difference in sex — for example, some women feel intimidated by male doctors/nurses, and some men are dismissive of female doctors/nurses.[11,19]

It may also be the case that the client can have difficulty communicating because of mental confusion, illness, tiredness, pain, emotional disease, lack of concentration or lack of a sense of self-worth. It is also possible that clients may exhibit considerable skills in defending his/her integrity and may be accomplished in manipulating the nurse and the interaction. Nurses should be aware of the social skills used in an interaction and the difficulties of employing such skills as listening or questioning.[20] However, the efforts of the client in listening and the emotional exertion it takes to reflect on feelings or discuss emotive issues may not always be recognised. How often is it acknowledged that treatment may be as tiring for the client as well as for the staff, and the client may be expending considerable energy in being pleasant or in exposing himself/herself to the treatment? This reinforces the value in developing skills in questioning and reflection of feelings.

The following section provides examples of various forms of questions, including recall, affective and process questions, and these may be used to enhance the communication process.

Questions: main types

There are three main types of questions: recall, affective and process.

Recall questions

These are used in order to obtain information from the client, and they may relate to personal details, dates, or events. These questions are often used at the beginning of an interview as a warm-up and to help the client relax. Examples of recall questions are:

'When was your operation?'
'Have you been to the clinic?'
'How many children have you?'

Recall questions are used for the interviewer to obtain facts; the interviewee is involved in giving information not exploring behaviour or attitudes.

Affective questions

This type of questioning is used in order for the interviewee to express opinions, preferences and feelings. Examples of affective questions are:

'What do you like about your job?'
'Are you afraid of the operation?'
'Do you feel lonely at times?'

Many of these questions can be followed by asking 'Why'.[21]

Process questions

Process questions are used when you want the interviewee to use his/her own knowledge and ideas in order:

(a) to give reasons or explanations;
(b) to make judgements or comparisons;
(c) to evaluate and analyse information;
(d) to make generalisations.

Sometimes doing this helps clarify the problem and can be therapeutic. This type of questioning helps the interviewer to gain understanding of the client; examples are:

'Why do you become angry at work?'
'What would you really like to happen?'
'In what way has this helped you?'
'What can you do about your stress?'

Closed and open questions

Questions can be closed or open.

Closed questions are those which require short factual answers, often one word, for example:

'Do you smoke?'
'What is your age?'

These kind of questions are suitable for information, but are not the best way of encouraging the interviewee to talk. For example, if you ask 'Are you feeling all right?', you will get a yes/no answer, but if you ask 'How are you feeling?', you will get a more illuminating answer.

Open questions are those which do not restrict the answer and which let the client talk around the area; examples are:

'How did you get on with your exercise last week?'
'What happened at the clinic yesterday?'
'What do you like best about coming here?'

Biased questions

There is also the danger of asking loaded or biased questions. For example, in the question 'Have you stopped beating your dog?', whether the answer is 'yes' or 'no' then you are guilty of cruelty.

Biased questions often indicate the answer that is expected, therefore the client is led to answer in a way which is thought desirable; examples are:

'I am sure you found that easy'
'You are feeling better, aren't you?'
'Are you really going to do that?'

Bias can also be present in asking about emotive topics when there is a pressure to answer in a socially accepted way.[22] Therefore to ask a mother 'Are you enjoying your baby?' will probably get a 'yes' because it would be difficult to answer in the negative. In this situation it might be better to say 'Sometimes new mothers feel under stress with a new baby — do you feel like that?' If you state the issue it makes it easier to get a more honest answer.

Clients will often want to please and will not wish to go against what is socially accepted, or thought to be the beliefs of the interviewer.

Dual questions

When asking questions it is easy to fall into the trap of asking more than one and so confusing the client who will not know which question to answer; examples are:

'Are you on your diet and what about the smoking?'
'Is this why you came — have you had it for long?'
'How do you sleep, what time do you go to bed?'

Keeping questions simple

Always try not to use jargon or difficult words when asking questions. This may seem very obvious, but the words and ideas nurses may take for granted are not in common usage and there may also be cultural differences in languages which hinders communication.

Questions are used to elicit feedback, to make sure the client has understood the message.[23] This can be difficult as you do not want to embarrass the client if he/she has not understood. Therefore it is best to use yourself in the question, for example:

'I am not sure I have explained this fully, could you tell me what I have to do?'
'In case I have missed out anything important could you just go over the main points again.'

If you simply ask: 'Have you understood', you will probably receive a 'yes' because the client is afraid to appear stupid.

Paralanguage and paraphrasing

Clients often need to be encouraged to continue talking, and the nurse can either do this by paralanguage such as 'mm mmm' or by saying 'I see', 'yes', 'that's interesting', 'tell me more', 'what happened then', 'great', 'that's a good point'.

Nurses can also use the skill of paraphrasing. This is a response to the client which states the main points of what is being said using the nurses' own words together with key words and phrases from the client; an example is: 'So you are not really sure about going on the pill'.

Dealing with emotions: reflection of feeling

The client may be expressing feelings about his/her situation and may be angry or sad or crying. It is often very difficult for a nurse to deal with such a display of emotion; but it is essential that she does. The main skill used in this type of situation is reflection of feeling, which is mirroring back to the client's verbal statements, to convey the feeling she/he is trying to communicate.[24] It is necessary to listen for words about feeling and to observe the non-verbal communication, for example:

'You seem worried about this pain.'
'You are very distressed by his behaviour.'

Reflecting meaning is the joining together of feelings and content in order to help explain what is happening, for example:

'You feel . . . because . . ..'
'You are disappointed . . . about . . ..'
'You feel good that you have managed to stop smoking.'
'You have difficulty with your mother because of her illness.'

CONCLUSIONS

Because of criticism of the way nurses communicate with patients,[25] there is an increasing emphasis on introducing social skills into training by providing distance learning materials.[26]

For much of the time, communication between nurse and client/patient is at a superficial level and is geared towards giving and receiving information or the exchange of pleasantries. The nurse has many opportunities during a working day to engage in communication at a deeper level. If such communication does not always take place, it could be that it is not actively encouraged by senior staff. It could also be that not everyone has the ability to communicate at this level, but such skills can be learned. It is a sad reflection on his/her stay in hospital that the patient can say, 'I was very well cared for, but the only people I could really talk to were other patients.' Nurses sometimes make it very plain to patients when their verbal approaches are unwelcome. The way the nurse moves swiftly from bed to bed, giving the impression of controlled haste, is enough to deter most people from trying to establish communication at anything other than a superficial level.[27] Conversation between staff and patients may be kept deliberately superficial by such techniques as joking, laughter and banter. These avoidance techniques, which may be unconscious, are a way of ensuring that deeper feelings are not readily available to be discussed.

By using non-verbal aspects of behaviour the nurse can convey to clients that she is interested in them and is keen to help in any way possible. The skilled nurse will make the session pleasurable, helped by a friendly smile, relaxed manner and an approach which is supportive without being threatening or demeaning. There are two important points worth stressing: first, people want to be with others who make them feel good; and second, to be interested in someone is the highest compliment you can pay them.

Within complementary therapies the underlying principle of 'holism' centres upon an interdependence of the mind, body and spirit by focusing upon the communication process using touch, close proximity to the patient, and verbal communication. It is a known fact that successful interaction between therapist and client can help to enhance the treatment given.

With orthodox nursing and health care, it has been argued that effective communication and social skills take time — a commodity in short supply in many nursing environments today, due to reduced staffing levels and increased workloads. Successful communication may not necessarily be dependent upon the *amount* of time staff spend with patients, but rather *how* that time is spent. In this respect the successful application of effective social skills should also greatly enhance the treatment given by orthodox nursing care.

In conclusion, a knowledge of social skills is not only valuable to staff involved in complementary therapies, but should also be interpreted as a fundamental tenet of any nursing and medical care given to patients.

REFERENCES

1. Hargie, O., Saunders, C. and Dickson, D. *Social Skills in Interpersonal Communication*. (Croom Helm, London, 1987).
2. Becker, H. 'Whose Side are We On?'. *Social Problems* (1967), 14, p. 24.
3. Stuart, G. and Sundeen, S. *Principles and Practice of Psychiatric Nursing*. (C.V. Mosby, St Louis, 1979).
4. Wiedenback, E. and Falls, C.E. *Communication Key to Effective Nursing*. (Triesias Press, New York, 1968).
5. Argyle, M. *Bodily Communications*. (Methuen, London, 1975).
6. Shapiro, J.G. 'Responsivity to Facial and Linguistic Cause'. *Journal of Communication* (1968), 18, pp. 11–17.
7. Morris, D. *Manwatching*. (Cape, London, 1978).
8. Nurse, G. *Counselling and the Nurse*. (HM and M, Aylesbury and John Wiley, Chichester, 1980).
9. Argyle, M. *The Psychology of Interpersonal Behaviour*. (Penguin, London, 1973).
10. Dickson, A. *A Woman in her Own Right*. (Penguin, London, 1982).
11. Ewels, L. and Simnet, I. *Promoting Health*. (John Wiley and Sons, Chichester, 1985).
12. Hall, E. *The Silent Language*. (Doubleday, New York, 1939).
13. Borck, L.E. and Fawcett, S.B. *Learning Counselling Problem-Solving Skills*. (Haworth Press, New York, 1982).
14. Argyle, M. (ed.) *Social Skills and Health*. (Methuen, London, 1981).
15. Bradley, J.C. *Communication in the Nursing Context* (Prentice-Hall, New York, 1982).
16. Egan, G. *The Skilled Helper*. (Brooks-Cole, Monterey, California, 1980).
17. Health Education Council (HEC) Training for Health and Race *Providing Effective Health Care in a Multiracial Society*. (Training for Health and Race, London, 1984).
18. Altschul, A. *Patient–Nurse Interaction*. (Churchill Livingstone, Edinburgh, 1972).
19. Ley, P. 'Psychological Studies of Doctor–Patient Communication', in Rachman, S. (ed.) *Contributions to Medical Psychology*. (Pergamon Press, Oxford, 1977).
20. Long, L., Paradise, L.V. and Long, T.J. *Questioning: Skills for the Helping Process*. (Brooks-Cole, Monterey, California, 1981).
21. Cavanagh, M.E. *The Counselling Experience: Understanding and Living It*. (Brooks-Cole, Monterey, California, 1982).
22. Munro, E.A., Manthei, J.J. and Small, J.J. *Counselling: A Skills Approach*. (Methuen, Wellington, New Zealand, 1979).
23. Ley, P., Bradshaw, P.W., Eaves, D. and Walker, C.M. 'A Method for Increasing Patients' Recall of Information Presented by Doctors'. *Psychological Medicine* (1973), 3, 217–20.
24. Smith, V.M. and Bass, T.A. *Communication for the Health Care Team*. (Harper and Row, New York, 1982).

25. Thompson, T. *Communication for Health Professionals*. (Harper and Row, London, 1986).

26. Holland, S. 'Teaching Patients and Clients'. *Nursing Times* (1987), 83 (9), pp. 56–8.

27. Stewart, W. *Counselling in Nursing*. (Lippincott, London, 1983).

14

Iridology

Stephanie Downey

INTRODUCTION

Iridology is a method of diagnosis using the iris of the eye. It is based on the theory that the macrocosm is reflected in the microcosm. This is a concept shared with other complementary medicines, for example reflexology and auricular therapy where the feet and the ears respectively represent, in microcosm, the entire body. In the case of iridology, a complex interrelationship between different parts of the body is recognised, so that any abnormality or malfunction is seen to be reflected in the iris. The aim of iridology is to identify precise areas of imbalance in the body which may not be accessible by conventional diagnostic methods since disease often originates far away from where the symptoms manifest. By seeing the 'whole person' through the iris, iridology provides great insight into the underlying causes, so that appropriate changes can be made to prevent further degeneration.

HISTORY

Iridology is essentially an empirical approach, founded on years of observation and correlation. It originated in Europe in 1881 with a Hungarian neurologist, Dr Ignatz von Péczely. When a young boy he found an owl and accidentally broke one of its legs, suddenly noticing a black line moving from the bottom of the bird's eye to the centre.[1] He watched the line gradually disappear as the leg healed. From this observation Dr von Péczely, in later years, began to note certain patterns in his patient's eyes. For example, those with lung problems often had dark spots in a specific part of their irises, and similarly those with stomach complaints often had grey or white rings around the pupils. This marked the beginning of the European School of Iridology which continued to be developed primarily by physicians in Germany, where it is now routinely practised by homeopathic doctors (p. 7).[1]

In America over 50 years ago a chiropractor, Dr Bernard Jensen, formulated a more simplified style of iris diagnosis. This was based on research done in Europe, but much less complex and less medically refined. Because of its greater accessibility to those who have no medical training, Jensen's work has widely become the definitive version for most iridology practitioners who work within complementary medicine.

THE THEORY OF IRIDOLOGY

It is impossible here to give more than a brief outline of the principles and practice of iris diagnosis. I would recommend that anyone wishing to understand iridology in greater depth refer to the bibliography and further reading list at the end of the chapter.

So, what can the iris tell us?

In general terms it is possible to determine the strength of someone's constitution, where their inherited weaknesses are, and whether they are causing any problems. More specifically, the iris reflects the state of the circulation and lymphatic system, the location of acute and chronic illnesses and the presence of accumulated toxins in the body.

An ideal iris will be a clear colour, either blue, grey or brown with no other unnatural colourings. The state of the fibres are a good indication of constitutional strength. These are the fine filaments which radiate out from the pupil to the iris edge, and ideally should be straight and densely packed. The tighter the fibres the stronger the body is and the better its healing ability (p. 72).[1]

Divisions of the iris

In order to 'read' the iris in detail, it is divided up into concentric zones radiating out from the pupil (Figure 14.1). These zones represent the general levels at which problems may occur.

Figure 14.1: Zones of the Iris

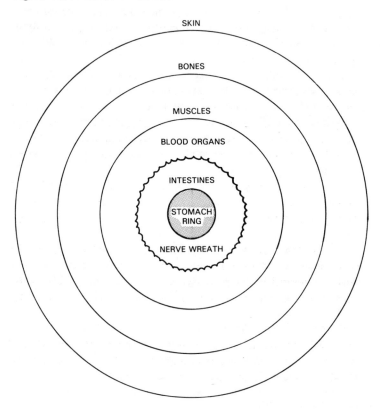

The innermost zones

The two innermost zones refer to the digestive organs, stomach and intestines. This is one of the most important areas since problems here can spill out into other parts of the body. Brown or dark coloration is an indication of bad diet, too much processed and over-refined food, leading to an unhealthy build-up of uneliminated toxic waste that may spread out to affect muscles, lymphatics, circulation and the skin. The stomach ring directly encircles the pupil, indicating different problems according to its colour. A white ring suggests hyperacidity, a grey one underactivity of the stomach, and a red brown ring suggests toxic poisoning of the gastric nerves (pp. 85–6).[1]

Nerve wreath

About one-third of the way out from the pupil to the iris edge is the 'nerve wreath'. This can easily be seen as a slightly jagged circle or ruff around the digestive zone. It represents the autonomic and central nervous system and the nerve supply to all the organs. Much can be diagnosed according to the shape and colour of the nerve wreath, which should have a uniform edge and be neither too close, nor too far away from the pupil. If it is very narrow and close to the pupil this indicates a sensitive constitution, and outpouchings into other areas are suggestive of gastrointestinal problems. A very ragged nerve wreath may mean some nervous system damage (p. 84).[1]

A regular nerve wreath in the correct place shows the ideal physical balance between contraction and relaxation of the body via the physical nerve fibres down the spine to all parts of the body (pp. 184–8).[2]

Points of tension in the body show up as outward peaks of the nerve wreath or contractions inwards. According to the exact location of abnormal markings in the nerve wreath (dark spots, white lines, yellow/brown colouring) very precise diagnoses can be made.

Third and fourth zones

The third and fourth zones represent the organs of transport and utilisation, plus elimination through the kidneys. These include blood and lymph vessels and the muscular system.

Fifth and sixth zones

The last two zones reflect the organs and structural support system, the bones and the skin. This outer area also indicates the body's ability to eliminate toxins and waste products (p. 16).[3]

Jensen's iris chart

The actual positions of individual organs and physiological systems are shown in Jensen's iris chart (Figure 14.2). As in a clockface, the exact location of an organ is described in hours and minutes. For example, the thyroid gland is at half past two in the right iris.

The right side of the body is represented in the right iris, and the left side by the left iris. This can sometimes be seen in terms of wear and tear on the body; for example, a right-handed person who constantly overuses one side of the body may show more signs of

Figure 14.2: Iris Map (a) Right eye, looking at another person's right eye. (b) Left eye, looking at another person's left eye

(a)

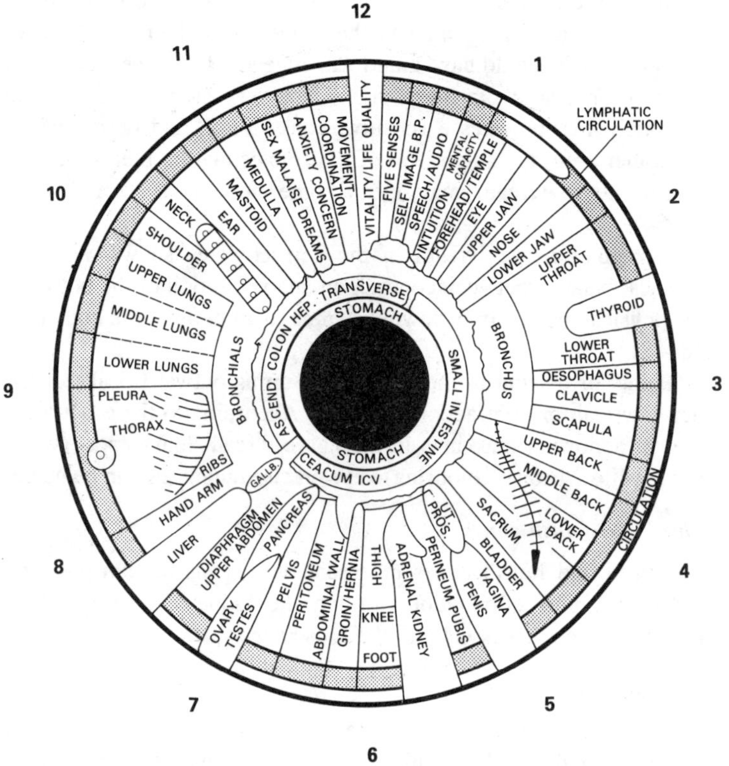

Iris map (b) left eye, looking at another person's left eye.

(b)

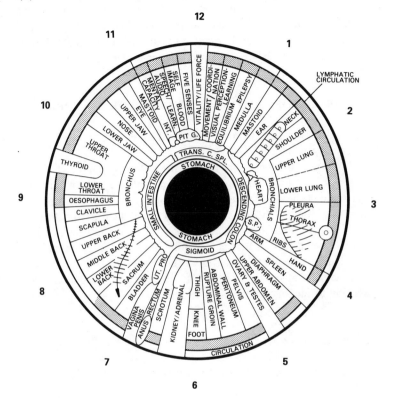

misaligned muscles and bones in the right iris (p. 17).[2]

This representation of the body in the iris map is not totally random; when studied carefully a certain logic emerges, for instance the top part of the body, the head, and mental processes are located at the top of the iris, while the pelvis, lower abdomen, legs and feet are at the bottom. Internal organs are nearer the pupil, and the more structural and superficial parts are nearer to the iris edge (p. 90).[2]

ABNORMALITIES AND WHAT TO LOOK FOR IN AN IRIS

Given that most people do not have ideal irises, how do we set about diagnosing what might be wrong?

First of all it is necessary to have the following: an iris chart (see Figure 14.2), a magnifying glass, and a pen torch. The magnifying glass should be held directly in front of the eye and the pen torch at an angle behind the glass. It is best to 'read' the iris from the pupil outwards and look at the general state of health and constitution to get an overall picture first before going into specific abnormalities. For example, look at the quality of the fibres, the colour of the iris and the state of the nerve wreath to provide a basic context before starting to identify particular markings.

Abnormal signs

(1) Unnatural colouring, shades of yellow, orange or brown.
(2) Dark spots.
(3) White or dark lines or 'spokes'.
(4) Holes known as lacunae.
(5) Wisps and clouds.
(6) Circular rings in or around the iris.

By relating the location of any of the above to the iris map, very specific diagnoses can be made according to their position in the iris. Here is a brief summary of some common abnormalities:

Brown spots or dark spots

These usually indicate an accumulation of toxins possibly due to medication, drugs or chemicals deposited in the tissues, which can either be inherited or accumulated through one's lifestyle and diet.

White lines and radiating spokes

These generally mean overstimulation and increased activity, whereas dark lines refer to insufficient stimulation or underactivity. For example, a white line over the spine may mean acute inflammation and pain, where darker lines here indicate a more chronic condition. Lines coming out from the stomach ring to the brain area would make one suspect headaches caused by gastric problems. These spokes radiating from the intestinal area are very common signs of toxicity, where the byproducts of the colon are contaminating other parts of the body.

Lacunae

Where straight lines in the iris refer to one particular organ, circular 'holes' in the fibres indicate a more generalised effect on the body. Lacunae appear as lesions where the iris fibres have pulled apart revealing a secondary layer. The severity of a lacuna is judged by its colour and depth (p. 75),[1] which indicate varying degrees of functional weakness and tissue degeneration.

Lacunae can, however, heal up and eventually become patched over as appropriate steps are taken to reverse the degeneration process. One of the most interesting things about the iris is its ability to reflect changes in the body, both before and after treatment.

Wisps and clouds

Strings of white spots around the periphery of the iris are known as the lymphatic rosary. This indicates an overburdened lymphatic system often related to allergies and problems digesting the proteins in milks and wheat. Common manifestations, especially when these marks occur in the facial area, are sinusitis, hay fever, catarrh or asthma.

Rings

A blue haze on the sclera around the iris or a fuzzy brown iris edge is often a sign of anaemia. Dark rings on the edge of the iris can indicate various accumulations of minerals in the body such as excess salt, magnesium, copper lead or mercury poisoning (pp. 98–103).[2]

Dark rings round the iris edge also reflect problems in the skin zone. The skin is seen as an organ of elimination helping rid the body of metabolic waste, so rings here often occur in people with eczema or psoriasis.

Transparent rings of 'crimped' fibres are known as stress or

227

nerve rings and directly relate to levels of stress in different parts of the body and the ability to relax.

For a more detailed description of how these markings form the basis of diagnosis see Kriege, chapters 8–20.[3]

RESEARCH

No one really knows how iridology works. Maxwell[1] suggests that the iris monitors the same bioelectric energy that acupuncture (p. 11) does.[1] She proposes that the basis for this phenomenon is the neuro-optic reflex, which '. . . turns the iris into an organic Etch-a-Sketch that monitors impressions from all over the body as they come in' (p. 11).[1]

Most of the research into iridology has taken place in Germany where it is still being developed and refined. As a form of complementary medicine it is relatively unknown in this country, and given little if any credence in orthodox medical circles. Iridology faces the same problems as do most other complementary therapies, the fact that it is not measurable in traditional 'scientific' terms. Until more 'holistic' research methods have been devised and accepted by the orthodoxy, iridology will remain on the fringe, its value dismissed merely as anecdotal evidence.

IRIDOLOGY FOR NURSES AND HEALTH PRACTITIONERS

As a non-invasive diagnostic method, iridology has potentially a wide area of application within the health field. Although it focuses purely on observable changes within the iris, iridology is essentially holistic since it recognises the effects of physical, emotional and environmental influences on the body, and hence the iris. The main strength of iridology is its ability to look beyond the symptoms and identify areas of disharmony that are closer to the real cause of the problem.

One example of how emotional signs can be diagnosed through the iris could be shown through someone who had a brown spot, or dull fog over the spleen area (left iris 4–5 o'clock). This may relate to suppressed spleen function due to an inability to release anger, or to show the kind of aggressive response and self-defence under attack that is necessary for survival. The actual physical symptoms of this low spleen function could range from low immunity or pathological tiredness to glandular fever or leukaemia (p. 205).[2] However, one of the most important rules of iridology is always to look at the *whole* context in which the person is operating. No iris sign can be interpreted in isolation. As Kriege points out 'one must always bear in mind that the eye represents a unity, and should be considered in its entirety' (p. 86).[3]

Therefore, to make a diagnosis using iridology it is important to take a full case history of present and past complaints, diet, lifestyle and emotional factors, and relate all interpretations to the individual's personal experience.

Iridology supports natural methods of healing based on nutrition, natural foods, herbs, fasting, exercise and rest, as only these will trigger classic healing signs in the iris. Drugs leave toxic residues which appear in the iris as unnaturally coloured flecks. Also, as Maxwell points out, drugs merely suppress the symptoms while they do nothing to correct the underlying causes (p. 11).[1]

The aim of iridology is to promote self-help mainly in the form of dietary changes. Cleansing diets with the elimination of meat, sugar and refined foods may often be recommended. Iridology also encourages an awareness of the damaging effects of certain emotional and environmental influences, so where possible changes can be made in these areas as well.

Iridology is commonly practised alongside some other form of natural therapy such as herbalism, homeopathy or naturopathy, and provides a valuable adjunct to back up other methods of diagnosis. However, it also has much to offer orthodox medicine especially in the area of preventive medicine.

For example, health visitors and school medical staff working with children could use iridology to detect the potential for ill-health and help prevent it through nutritional, environmental, and psychological advice.

By observing preclinical signs, appropriate steps can be taken to prevent a disease from manifesting, and even if symptoms are present iridology can monitor an improvement in health.

Unfortunately nurses working with the constraints of hospital regulations, where their role is more strictly defined, have less opportunity to practise complementary therapies such as iridology. While doctors make the diagnoses and order the treatment, it is difficult for nurses to find the autonomy necessary to carry out more holistic approaches to patient care.

District nurses have more freedom in this sphere, since their patients are not subject to such rigorous medical intervention, and she can usually work more on her own initiative. Also the insights a district nurse may have into her patient's personal and domestic life will enable her to practise a broader, more preventive form of therapy. Iridology is something that everyone can be taught to use both on others and themselves. Patients may be taught the principles of iris diagnosis to provide self care, monitor changes in their own health, and maintain optimum health with minimum intervention. This similarly applies to health practitioners in the way they look after their own health. All that is needed to 'read' your own eyes is a mirror and a reverse iridology chart, which shows a mirror image of the one illustrated in Figure 14.2.

Although a thorough training is required to make the complex and refined diagnoses necessary in professional practice, the basics of iridology can be easily learnt. Because of this, it is of immense value for those who wish to use it among friends and family, to bring a greater awareness of the body's warning signs and its ability for self-healing.

CONCLUSIONS

Iridology is not well understood and consequently has a long way to go before it is widely accepted. It is not an absolute diagnostic method and therefore must be applied carefully to avoid gross generalisation through lack of awareness of the 'whole person'.

However, increasing evidence in both Europe and the United States continues to support the early observations made by German physicians over 100 years ago. As more research is done the value of iridology will be increasingly recognised as an easily accessible diagnostic method that promotes good health through natural processes.

REFERENCES

1. Maxwell, J. *The Eye/Body Connection*. (Warner Books, New York, 1980).
2. Hall, D. *Iridology*. (Angus and Robertson, London, 1980).
3. Kriege, T. *Fundamental Basis of Iris Diagnosis*. (L.N. Fowler, Essex, UK, 1980).

BIBLIOGRAPHY AND FURTHER READING

See references above.

USEFUL ADDRESSES

British School of Iridology
Bright Haven
Robin's Lane
Lolworth
Cambridge
CB3 8HH
Telephone: 0954 81074

National Council and Register of Iridologists
Lacnunda
80 Portland Road
Bournemouth
BH9 1NQ
Telephone: 0202 529793
(Information on registered iridologists, courses and seminars)

Index